T0235919

AUTOBIOGRAPHY OF A DISEASE

Autobiography of a Disease documents, in experimental form, the experience of extended life-threatening illness in contemporary US hospitals and clinics. The narrative is based primarily on the author's sudden and catastrophic collapse into a coma and long hospitalization thirteen years ago; but it has also been crafted from twelve years of research on the history of microbiology, literary representations of illness and medical treatment, cultural analysis of MRSA in the popular press, and extended autoethnographic work on medicalization.

An experiment in form, the book blends the genres of storytelling, historiography, ethnography, and memoir. Unlike most medical memoirs, told from the perspective of the human patient, *Autobiography of a Disease* is told from the perspective of a bacterial cluster. This orientation is intended to represent the distribution of perspectives on illness, disability, and pain across subjective centers—from patient to monitoring machine, from body to cell, from caregiver to cared-for—and thus makes sense of illness only in a social context.

Patrick Anderson is Associate Professor in the departments of Communication, Ethnic Studies, and Critical Gender Studies at the University of California, San Diego. He is the author of *So Much Wasted* and the co-editor (with Jisha Menon) of *Violence Performed*.

Writing Lives

Ethnographic Narratives

Series Editors: Arthur P. Bochner, Carolyn Ellis and Tony E. Adams
University of South Florida and *Northeastern Illinois University*

Writing Lives: Ethnographic Narratives publishes narrative representations of qualitative research projects. The series editors seek manuscripts that blur the boundaries between humanities and social sciences. We encourage novel and evocative forms of expressing concrete lived experience, including autoethnographic, literary, poetic, artistic, visual, performative, critical, multi-voiced, conversational, and co-constructed representations. We are interested in ethnographic narratives that depict local stories; employ literary modes of scene setting, dialogue, character development, and unfolding action; and include the author's critical reflections on the research and writing process, such as research ethics, alternative modes of inquiry and representation, reflexivity, and evocative storytelling. Proposals and manuscripts should be directed to abochner@usf.edu, cellis@usf.edu or aeadams3@neiu.edu

Other volumes in this series include:

Evocative Autoethnography
Writing Lives and Telling Stories
Arthur P. Bochner and Carolyn Ellis

Bullied
Tales of Torment, Identity, and
Youth
Keith Berry

**Collaborative and Indigenous
Mental Health Therapy**
Tataihono – Stories of Maori
Healing and Psychiatry
*Wiremu NiaNia, Allister Bush and
David Epston*

For a full list of titles in this series, please visit: www.routledge.com/Writing-Lives-Ethnographic-Narratives/book-series/WLEN

AUTOBIOGRAPHY OF A DISEASE

Patrick Anderson

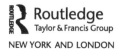

Routledge
Taylor & Francis Group

NEW YORK AND LONDON

First published 2017
by Routledge
711 Third Avenue, New York, NY 10017

and by Routledge
2 Park Square, Milton Park, Abingdon, Oxon, OX14 4RN

Routledge is an imprint of the Taylor & Francis Group, an informa business

© 2017 Taylor & Francis

Library of Congress Cataloging in Publication Data
Names: Anderson, Patrick, 1974– author.
Title: Autobiography of a disease / Patrick Anderson.
Description: New York, NY : Routledge, 2017. | Series: Writing lives: ethnographic narratives
Identifiers: LCCN 2016058684| ISBN 9781138744486 (hbk) | ISBN 9781138744509 (pbk) | ISBN 9781315180991 (ebk)
Subjects: LCSH: Staphylococcus aureus infections. | Methicillin resistance.
Classification: LCC RC116.S8 A53 2017 | DDC 616.9/2–dc23
LC record available at https://lccn.loc.gov/2016058684

ISBN: 978-1-138-74448-6 (hbk)
ISBN: 978-1-138-74450-9 (pbk)
ISBN: 978-1-315-18099-1 (ebk)

Typeset in Bembo
by Wearset Ltd, Boldon, Tyne and Wear

For my mother,
and mothers everywhere,
in whatever form they take.
And for Kaja.

Identity exists where the Complication and Unraveling are the same.

Aristotle, *The Poetics*

This then is life,
Here is what has come to the surface
after so many throes and convulsions.

Walt Whitman, *Leaves of Grass*

CONTENTS

FOREWORD

Sometime during the fall of 2003—I'm still not sure exactly when—I fell suddenly and violently ill. Within hours, I was unconscious. And when I awoke—I'm still not sure exactly when—the world, and my place in it, had dramatically changed. Over the course of the year and more that followed, as a wide variety of doctors and nurses sought first to diagnose and then to prognosticate over the cause of my collapse, I found myself deeply immersed in an accidental ethnography of what goes by the name of "care" in contemporary US medical practice: endless imaging technologies, documentary protocols, interventional procedures and surgeries, occupational training, independent living schemes, and countless other social practices gathered under the headings "convalescence" and "recovery." Trained both as an anthropologist and as a performance scholar, I slowly realized that, like it or not, I had stumbled into what became an extraordinarily intricate and complex research field: the practice of dying, or nearly, and getting "well."

But awakening in the midst of an illness that treads precariously at the precipice of mortality is never a singular event, nor is it linear in its progression. Over the course of that year spent in hospitals, my apprehension of what was happening to and around me was shaped and distorted by fluctuating states of consciousness, pain drugs and anesthetics, dreams and hallucinations, rapid cycles of recovery and deterioration, and by the shifting tides of interactions with the many people entrusted with caring for me. I wanted to know and understand what was happening—both for my own sake, and out of anthropological curiosity—but I could not depend upon my own capacity for knowing or understanding. What in one moment might seem clear would, on the following day or with the next procedure, dissemble itself into fiction or myth. I looked to others—"interlocutors," in the anthropological vernacular—to explain what was happening, what had happened, what it meant. I learned, as Tim Parks has written, that "every illness is a narrative," and that "what matters is the version you tell yourself."[1]

This book is about illness. But it is also about how we make sense of being-ill. As an ethnography, it is founded upon multiple kinds of research over the last ten years: archival study of the origins of microbiology, diagnosis, and treatment protocols; reviews of medical, popular, and media literature about drug-resistant bacterial strains; exhaustive reading and re-reading of (my own) patient records and medical files; and, of course, interviews with medical professionals, patients, and caregivers. But it also acknowledges that understanding the experience of illness exceeds even these dependable academic methodologies. And so this book takes something of a radical leap: it distributes the agency of narration—the power to describe—not just to the many human actors involved in treatment and care-taking, but also to the non-sentient beings involved in the practice of being-ill. How do microbes understand the human diseases they sometimes occasion? How does a discarded fragment of human bone tissue remember (or mourn) its former function? How do damaged retinal tissue and visual receptors in the brain make sense of the fractured images they collect? Can an EKG take pleasure in the rhythms it records?

This book, then, understands illness not as a patient's monologue or biography, but as a profoundly social, richly durational, and multiply perspectival encounter. It seeks to describe how illness makes meaning of the world even as it threatens to dissemble the world in which it occurs. The structure of the narrative that follows is episodic and, at times, disjointed; but it nonetheless follows a timeline of illness as experienced by those who were gathered in its sweep. The soul of its intent—to describe and understand a series of events that occurred in a particular sociocultural context—overlaps with recent trends in a number of academic discourses (including autoethnography, medical humanities, distributed cognition, disability studies, and performance studies). But it also exceeds those designations, seeking to embrace the constant stream of disorientation, misrecognition, and radical undoing that occupies the very heart of illness's ontology; it is to such crises that push the limits of knowing and knowability that this book bears witness.

Note

1 Tim Parks, *Teach Us to Sit Still: A Skeptic's Search for Health and Healing* (New York: Rodale, 2012), 27.

PRELUDE

What it was we had to tell him couldn't have been said in whispers, shouts, or sighs, but only in the ancient tongue of death, of falling sick and dying young. What it was we had to tell him had been haunting us for years, a nagging voice in the back of our own minds, like the most guttural sob or the heartiest of belly-laughs, like newborn hair, like wind after rain, like a sunset in smog, like an egg: perfect and perfectly clear. What it was we had to tell him we could not ourselves understand, not in the way that he would; it was a message from a cause to the victim of an effect. We did not mind that it was ours to tell him. We only prolonged the telling because it felt so good to know that we had not told him yet. We have so very little to look forward to.

But we begin with the story of our origins, of our own halting starts in the world. We were born of a resolute mother. Her voice was chewed by cigarettes and whiskey, or so it would seem to those of you who have access to the domain of sound. She is a tiny thing, and if everyone calls her "the little terror" it is only because such strength rarely comes in packages as small as her. She prowls the routes and ways to which she has access with a hunger satiable only by multiplication: the sense we sometimes get that others are becoming more and more like us, the sense that the world is conforming to our singular notion of what it should be, the sense that we grow larger by convincing others that there is no other way but ours.

And she has never been defeated—not really, though her form has changed dramatically over the years. This is her greatest defense: a mutability the Greeks personified and named Morpheus, a name ironically recognizable now in the chemicals that provide fleeting release from the pain our mother can cause. She responds to threat with the ultimate bait-and-switch, modulating her slow, sinuous assault just enough to avoid any reactionary blows. She knows her itinerary well, though, and does not waver from it. Her object is life, her aim is expansion, and her method is to sneak unseen—or without raising an alarm—through whatever back doors she can find.

Her name isn't easy on the tongue. Some call her Mersa, a lyrical name, a name that sings; but she prefers the longer version: Methicillin Resistant Staphylococcus Aureus. She likes to say—or would if she could—that hearing it makes her proud. This is a complicated pride. The first word in her name was shared by a lover who, like most lovers, ended up breaking her heart and almost destroying her entirely. She once thought, like many maybe most, that this lover was destined for her, fashioned from the start as her perfect complement, that mythical other half for whom she had always been searching. And when that love failed, as love so often does, she thought that it was she herself—not her lover, not the pairing, not the circumstances through which they had found one another—who was flawed. The loss of love made her desperate to survive. The loss of faith in love made her determined to reinvent herself so that survival was no longer in question.

And in the years since that particular love failed, she has stretched out in so many directions that she is now only barely recognizable. Like a master linguist, her vocabularies of expansion are so vast, so subtly insistent, so treacherously unrelenting, that she rarely finds someone with whom she is unable to commune. Like empathy unchecked, she so gracefully moves from one station in life to another, that you might mistake her enthusiasm for kindness or concern. But just as this appetite for travel is not buoyed by an underlying compassion for those she does not know, neither is it driven by apathy, hatred, or greed. She is not a monster. Like most of us and maybe you, she is simply wounded, fragile in spite of her fortitude. It would be unbecoming, and somehow dishonest, for her to give up and pass away.

But if there is an outside to pain, our mother knows that place too. She dwells not only in the present, but also in the past: where memory retroactively becomes reality, where the trauma of suffering now is nothing more than an unknown future. She is devastatingly here, just as she always has been. But the story of her discovery is also the story of what you call progress, of knowledge giving birth to a cure, a "Eureka!" moment that changed (for better, for worse) centuries defined by the misunderstood meaning of life.

We can tell this story—what is essentially his, Patrick's, story—because we know it best, from the inside out, as it were. We are the branch of our mother's family tree that touched him, that invested him with unwanted significance, and that altered forever who he was and will have been. There are so many causes for illness, so very many etiologies of disease. Ours may be most base. We can take away your life, give you in greedy palms your final shudder and gasp, send you briefly but terrifically reeling through the final moments of the minuscule existence that defines what and who you are. We are that serious, and we are that strong. We have survived your many attempts to eradicate us, after all; and we know, better than you, how desperately you depend upon us to survive.

But when you attack—especially if you think you've won—you won't even see us coming, no matter how vigilant your attention. We do not arrive in images, but in the unspoken language of suffering. In short: we creep.

But the truth is that we come to depend upon you. In this case, it happened slowly. First we were there with him because he provided a safe place for us to be. Then, unwillingly perhaps, just out of trust for what the experts told him, he began to fight us, believing that we were all harm. And achingly, we grew stronger—learning the tricks of the tactics they used to hunt and eliminate us, dodging every bullet by the slightest of margins. We learned to be tenacious from our mother, and it took every gram of strength we had just to survive all that they threw at us. After a while, we realized that we were exactly what he needed, an insurrection in the deadening habits of daily life, a wake-up to his own vulnerability. We held our ground for his benefit as much as our own. And we dragged him forward, through the early phase more than the last, by pulling out from his memory-store other voices, other rooms; we dragged him forward by summoning visions, remembrances of his fractured past. This allowed us to work unhindered, even as we watched his flashbacks and dreams as if they were our own. We grew to care for him then, or started to, as we watched.

The love came later. It took us utterly by surprise.

PART I

1

He was abed for more than a week. It seemed like years—decades even—but in reality it couldn't have been more than a few months: a fall, winter, spring, early summer wasted with the business of getting well. His long, slow gasps; his murmured pleas for release from the pain that kept him fixed to the bed they'd pinned him to; his quick glances up to find that his mother—real or imagined he didn't know—was still hovering over him: these defined his days, as a tomcat defines the alley in which it prowls.

He awoke as if from a very deep sleep. The first time he awoke, it was to the image of his family. They were standing above his hospital bed, but in his haze they appeared to be in the front garden of a lush hotel. His father and step-mother stood, a fountain glimmering behind them, with arms interlocking. They looked askance, just off to the left of where he was sitting. His brothers and sister leaned in various postures around the green, looking at the sky, picking something off the ground, or smiling in some silent conversation. "Can you see us? Patrick, can you see us? Do you know we're here?" his stepmother said, her soft southern intonations the immediate comfort of, say, a stiff drink. "Jonathan, he can't see us."

His father, Jonathan, was silent, and looked clenched in seizure. Jonathan was the pastor of a small country church just off the Mississippi delta. He had a flair for the dramatic, but now his considerable talents at gesture and metaphor failed him. He was only here, now; the terrible stories of his childhood on an arid farm, typically boiling just beneath the surface, were miles or years away. There was only this: the sight of his oldest son—the son he idolized least, but understood most—lying on a gurney, surrounded and impaled by tubes, catheters, and IVs. There was only this. And he, Patrick, registering his father's presence in the periphery of his sightline, he began again to fall asleep.

"Keep," he started to say.

"What's that? Patrick? What did you say?" His father leaned closer.

"Keeping." This was all he could manage before he was out again, slipping farther away from that pleasant, almost comforting scene before the garden-mirage.

2

"No good will come of keepin' all this mess packed up in a box. Take what you want, and don't get ornery if somebody wants to take it from you somewhere down the line. Keepin's only good for givin'." Patrick's maternal grandmother, oozing Appalachia, murmured this one fall while they were looking together through her beat-up bridal trunk, now full of pictures—old photographs not sealed in frames or albums, just thrown into a makeshift pyre of people and places forgotten. He found a picture of his mother asleep on a bunk when she was fourteen. It was the only time he'd seen his mother sleeping. So he put the picture in his pocket, took it home, and hung it near his bed.

There was also, in that trunk, a picture of his mother at eighteen, the head majorette at her high school. She was all high boots with frills, tall pointy hat, arms akimbo in some pose as her baton spun twenty feet in the air and plunged back down to the crook of her elbow. She was all south Florida high school diva with a tan, white blonde hair, and sass like nobody's business. When he was a kid, and his parents were still embroiled in their bitter, ridiculous marriage, they lived in a cramped apartment for years. Then they lived in a house. In the basement of this house was a tiny laundry room, the only room he and his brother were banned from entering. It was his mother's private retreat, and she would spend hours there with the door closed, folding sheets and socks and shirts. Patrick would sneak up to the door when it was closed, and listen to her as she faintly, faintly hummed some song he didn't know, or talked to herself, working out the intricacies of some conversation she was going to have with someone he'd never met. He would try to imagine what her life was like when she was away or the others weren't home. At the time, he thought she was a beauty queen. She was a princess. She was the face and body and soul of love. He wanted her to be his whole world, and the thought that she had her own life to lead worried him.

Hanging on the wall in the laundry room was a large round case, vinyl and old, with her name painted in fancy cursive across the top. They all knew it was some kind of secret, and they knew it hung there for a reason. One day he snuck in and opened it to find one of her favorite batons, the kind that's affixed to a hula-hoop. He wondered if she stared up at it while doing laundry, remembering what it was like to be eighteen, living on the beach, taunting all those south Florida boys with her dazzling routines and string bikinis. He wondered if she considered beating his father over the head with it, then taking the car and her baton and driving away forever. He wondered if, when they were away, she took it out to the backyard and practiced twirling it, spinning herself into a frenzy before turning to face her imaginary crowd with a Miss America smile, catching the baton just before it struck ground. What did this mean, he wondered when he was a kid. Did he have secrets too? Would he keep them until he was old? Would he die with them? And where could he get one of those batons?

When his mother left his father, she didn't beat the man over the head with her baton. She just drove to the other side of the city, leaving almost everything they'd collected together in that old house. She didn't want anything he'd ever touched, not the furniture, not her clothes, not his money, nothing. She did take Patrick, but she made him take a long shower before he got in the car. She also took that old round case, and she hung it in her room in their new apartment. It was the only thing on her walls for a while, until gradually it was surrounded by paintings of beaches and photographs of her new lover. It disappeared entirely one day, and he didn't see it again until ten years later, when he was visiting her in a new town and she was giving him things to take home. They played his grandmother's old game, sitting around the bridal trunk, looking at his baby blanket (the one with a forlorn football embroidered onto a corner), a toy doctor's kit he'd had as a kid, and pictures of their little family before the split. They looked miserable in those pictures—especially his mother, whose body seemed to be stuck in a permanent clench. At the end of the night, they found the baton case, stuck way back in a box somewhere. His mother grew quiet, looked at it for what seemed like a year. She unzipped it slowly, pulled out the hoop baton, and handed it to him. "You ever learn how to twirl one of these things?"

"Keepin's only good for givin'," she might have said; but at this point in her life, his mother had noticed how closely her body was beginning to mimic her mother's, and she was desperate to fend off any further resemblance. Instead she smiled, and left the baton with him as she took off for the graveyard shift. He was rocked by the sentimentality he'd never before seen in her. He felt, for once, *inside*—him: the kid forever trying to fit into cliques that wouldn't have him, learning over and over how to temper resentment with creativity, how to turn rejection into love.

3

The second time he awoke, the Unknowns were huddled over him, grouped up in an urgent conference, moving slowly like dancers. All he knew was that there was something down his throat: it sounded like rubber but felt like steel. Later he would learn that this was one of the many devices they used to track the bacteria's progress. In fact, when he awoke for that second time, they did not yet know that they were there, that they were the cause of his sudden collapse.

He did not respond to the shock of his position with anything more than a quick intake of breath (stifled, of course, by the device that blocked his airway) and a frantic looking-around. His eyes darted for an instant from left to right and back again, before settling comfortably, almost familiarly, on the Unknown closest to him. Within minutes, the sedative dripping into his veins was intensified, and he was asleep again.

The third time he awoke they were there again, the Unknowns, but now sticking needles in his eyes. This time he awoke with a start, and was paralyzed by what he saw: the Unknowns wearing machines strapped across their foreheads, ticking and humming like little living things from a science fiction film. These machines had eyes of their own: bright, bulbous lamps shining beams that seemed to cut directly into his brain. He felt someone gripping his hand as the needles were withdrawn. He heard a voice telling him not to move. He pulled against the straps tying his wrists to the bars of his bed. The Unknowns told him to turn his eyes to the left, and then to the right, and then towards the ceiling, and then towards his feet. He heard their silence at what they saw, and he knew there was no good news. Something was wrong.

He directed himself to think backwards, and was confronted with a very deep blank. He could remember nothing. He tried again, thought harder. And something began to materialize: a conversation with a friend. He was there, in his small apartment, sitting on an overstuffed couch. He was hungry. But every time he tried to stand and make his way into the kitchen, nausea swelled and he relaxed back into the cushions again. The telephone was ringing, and he could not reach it. It rang again. And then the knock on his door. He remembered turning to look, to see if he could will it to open. And remarkably it did. Someone was coming inside, someone he knew. She was smiling, calling his name. "Patrick?" He remembered his name. He thought about the sound of his name, tried saying it back to her to feel what it did on his tongue. He tried again; "Pat" was as far as he got before he noticed her again, saw that her face had fallen, her eyes were wide open—like a cat's, he thought, like a cat's eyes when hunting a toy. She was running from the door to the couch. She dropped something, and he laughed at the sound that it made on the floor: a clang, a silly splash like something out of a cartoon.

The Unknowns noticed he was smiling. They took this as a compliment, that they had managed to mask his pain with pills. One of them smiled back, said "Patrick. You're going to be all right. Just hold still." But he was miles away, and this voice never reached him. He was miles away, playing back those splashes and clangs, watching his friend run comically across the room, her face a caricature of concern. He slipped even further back, to the Saturday mornings of his childhood. He was never one for the new animation. His favorites were always the oldest cartoons—Mickey Mouse, Bugs Bunny—played like apologies on the television channels that couldn't really compete. He remembered the shag wool on the floor, more comfortable than his bed. He remembered the brick façade of the wall. He remembered the tiny screen in the corner of the room, set opposite the fireplace, dressed with a doily and silk flowers. Irises, he thought. They were irises.

"We've lost him." The third time he awoke, this was the last thing he heard before falling asleep again.

4

When Patrick was young, his mother's mother lived in a small town in North Carolina. Every year at Thanksgiving, his family would make the long drive from Birmingham to his grandmother's house, where they were treated like strange visiting royalty. As they drove through the Blue Ridge Mountains each November, he would watch out the window at the shapes the hills made against the darkening autumn sky, and wonder what kind of miracle it took to make them look like reclining bodies. They were immaculate, far more beautiful than anyone he had ever seen sleeping in real life, and they stood in sharp contrast to the lazy, rolling hills of Birmingham. These mountains hid secrets from the drivers who carelessly passed them by; and as the family car made its strained way slowly through their mysterious paths, his father would forget where he was, and hum or occasionally sing along with the station he had found on the radio tuner: Ink Spots, Lettermen, Shandrelles. The soundtrack for their slow ascent up into the Appalachians was doo-wop, unchained melodies, early R&B. They covered their ears with those sounds, peeking out from under the tin roof of the battered old Chevy, hoping they wouldn't be swallowed up into the endless forests and bottomless caves that make those mountains feel like exclusion and like home, all at once.

When they arrived, his mother's mother—though she had clearly been waiting for hours, possibly even days, in advance—would be making herself busy with some ordinary chore. Typically, her famous peanut butter cake would sit temptingly on the kitchen counter; his brother and he would sneak peeks and, when they were brave, short, fast tastes of its sinful icing. His grandmother had always been a collector, and every year she found some new icon to decorate her life: first it was lemons, then roses, then hummingbirds that shone proudly from the corners of kitchen towels and sat in repose on every window sill. The trick was to guess what she would pick next, and no one ever could. There was no logic in her movement across phyla and species, just a simple grace that shifted her attention, her love, from fruit to flower to beast.

His grandmother was also a nurse, a fierce one, who worked in the local hospital and, for a month each year, on the streets of Calcutta. She would return from India every spring with tiny gifts—sandalwood camels, brass frames, incense—and a box full of slides. These were his introduction to the world outside himself and to the world of travel: blurry images of brightly colored saris and dusty roads, ramshackle homes filled with grinning children, aerial shots of the dense cities of South Asia. What he felt while looking at those images, shining down from the wood-paneled wall of the dining room, was a kind of vertigo, his body spinning, spinning him out of itself, his eyes losing focus, his feet straining to reach the ground that gave them rest.

At the far end of his grandmother's kitchen was a forbidden door that had been nailed shut into its frame, and lined with bolts and chains that made opening it a horrible inevitability. The story of the door was this: long before his grandmother lived in this house, a second-story porch had been built off the kitchen, overlooking the verdant hills that surrounded the property. At some point, that porch had crumbled, but had never been rebuilt. What remained was this door that led nowhere—or rather, this door that led to the nowhere of a deep, dark fall and a painful collision with the unforgiving ground below. As kids, he and his brother used to tempt fate by prying at the door's edges, hoping for a glimpse of their own vertiginous deaths. Or they would hide in the woods outside, staring through the trees at the outer side of the door, which was somehow more terrifying than its inside face. They imagined the unfortunate others who must have come before them, who must have tripped through the door and fallen to their doom, who must now be staring back at them in their ghostly forms, tickling their goose-bumped skin with long, airy fingers and sickening, lanky toes. They'd run screaming back inside, begging for the relief of their grandmother's hugs and the medicine found only in an oversized slice of her unbelievably scrumptious cake.

That feeling of loss, the one that came tumbling into him when he peered at his grandmother's slides, and when he imagined his body slamming into the mud below that door, stayed with him, in its hidden form, long after he was a child, long after his grandmother moved from her quiet mountain house to an even quieter cabin on a tiny lake not twenty miles down the road. That feeling of loss, the one you can't even approach with words, became the source and the limit of all his fears, of all his deepest wants.

5

What unbridled passion it must have taken to build this town, where against all odds these buildings and streets pack a proud and angry slope that rises furiously from bay to peak. On certain days in December, in radical disregard for the supposed pure and simple perfection of this place, snow falls in the hills, reminding all who live here that they are visitors, not exactly welcome, and destined not to stay for long. On other days in September, the ground will shake with such vengeance that everything they've built shifts, if just an inch, as though settling into a long and fitful sleep. What oblivious peace it must take to settle here.

The fourth time he awoke he was alone, his bed turned towards a window that covered an entire east-facing wall. He could not see completely, not as he had before; and what he could see was blurred just enough to make the image seem flawless, made perfect by its indistinct and hazy lines. At first he was not sure what he was seeing: fever dreams had taken away his faith not only in his ability to look, but also in everything that presented itself to be looked upon. What just yesterday appeared to him as an evil, crouching man was now nothing more than a lazy sling-back chair; where before he saw the silhouettes of family members long-ago dead, he now saw shadows cast back to the wall through the yellow shade of a table lamp. He turned his eyes to the window, saw in fractured, blurry pieces the town he had come to call home. He faintly saw the flashing lights of afternoon traffic, playing urgently across the walls of his room. He saw the hills in the distance, their massive mansions hidden beneath the graceful reach of redwood and eucalyptus trees. He heard the scrambling voices of children being herded onto a bus. He felt the pressure to remember.

Later they told him that he would never remember it all, that what they called a side effect of his condition was to lose his grasp of what had happened, perhaps to recall certain details here and there, but never the story as a whole. Later it would occur to him that only those who barter in illness, but have never been ill themselves, could call amnesia a side effect. He had always had a sharp and agile memory. Losing it was probably the greatest loss of all.

But now, before he knew, as he lay in this bed and watched for a sign that someone else was here, he thought only of that scene outside, its faint light as night came, its sounds a gentle reminder that the world does indeed pass us by, its rolling motion a calm refusal to pretend that it even noticed he was there at all.

6

Patrick's mother, Deirdre, had no patience for texts. He held vague memories of her opening books with every good intention of reading them, of participating in some small way in the vast love of the written word that her oldest son had for so long felt. (She didn't know, or maybe she did, that this was a love defined by escape. Maybe she knew this intimately, and sought precisely the same kind of remove.) But she never got farther than the first few pages, bored with how still she had to remain in order to focus completely on whatever stories were being told. Her mind started to drift, her leg would shake, and before long she had forgotten what she had only just read. Closing the book, she would withdraw to her room, dress in her running clothes, and leave for hours of exercise.

Writing held a special kind of mystery for her, and was vaguely offensive. It was obscene, invasive even, to attempt to name and expose her expansive inner life. She was a runner, not a writer.

But she learned how to write. In the hours and days during which she watched her son gripped by belief in some far-away hallucination, Deirdre began to grow suspicious of the care the Doctors performed. Or rather, she began to believe that their tightly staged visitations were precisely opposite to care. But she was not by nature adversarial, and tended to play along with structures of authority, even as she resisted them with delicate diversions. This is the complicated choreography of southern personhood, where a soft-spoken "Thank you" may just as well mean "Die."

Late one night, unable to sleep in the uncomfortable chairs of the waiting room and unable to think of anything other than fear, she left to walk the sterile-smelling halls of the hospital, and eventually came upon another like herself—another woman, like herself, sitting outside an ailing son's room, staring with such intensity at the nurses' station that it might at any moment melt under the pressure of, to put it mildly, maternal concern.

"I don't think they're helping my son," she said to Deirdre.

This was the first time that anyone had given voice to what Deirdre herself had been feeling since she had been summoned to this place. And suddenly, like a boil that begins to express, her exhaustion, her profound sense of betrayal, and her alienating distrust of almost everything they'd said, came bursting forth with such overwhelming force that she collapsed into the arms of this stranger.

She wept.

The stranger held her as she longed to hold her son, who was too fragile to endure even an embrace: not tenderly, knowing intimately that Deirdre had had enough of tenderness, but pragmatically, to keep her from falling further to the floor. Then suddenly she said with the severity of a preacher:

"Write it down. You have to write it down. All of it."

Deirdre shifted uncomfortably into the chair beside the stranger. She looked at her hands, now her own mother's hands, thickly veined, pocked with the scars of survival, strong.

"I can't. I can't write rage."

The woman handed her a book, thick and worn, covered in what seemed an unknown language: numbers and graphs, long unpronounceable words, pictures of wounds.

"Not rage."

Deirdre began reading. The book was filled with hospital desiderata: temperature and blood pressure readings, quantities of pills and dosage times, the names of hypothesized conditions, medical license numbers, insurance contacts. She had chronicled weeks of her son's convalescence, a portrait in data of illness, but also an archive of not-knowing. Deirdre asked:

"Do you know what all of this means?"

"I have no idea. But neither do they."

"Why write it down?"

"It keeps me from having to remember. And a few times, I've stopped them from killing him. One of them tried to give him a shot he'd already had. Another one thought the tattoo of a circle on his back was drawn in preparation for a procedure he wouldn't have survived. Someone else called him 'Brian.' Brian, whoever he is, was due for Radiation. My son is David."

Deirdre turned back to the book. In the margins she saw small pictures drawn by an unstudied hand, surrounded by minor adjectives: deep, wet, sharp. The stranger pointed at them and said:

"That's my son's pain. They kept asking him to describe how much he hurt on a scale of one to ten. It was always a ten. They tried six different kinds of painkillers, not knowing which would work. Every time. Like a guessing game. I realized at some point that pain is the only thing David knows more than the Doctors. They can't measure it except by how he describes it—no machines, no thermometers, no X-ray can tell them how he hurts. Only his words. I helped him come up with these."

Dry, shallow, loud.

"Are they working?"

The woman turned back to stare at the Nurses' Station. "I don't know. He's having fever dreams again. He talks in his sleep about falling, sometimes about something chasing him. Sometimes he just shudders, like he's cold. They cover him in blankets." Her hands moved to her lap, a misleading mien of calm. "All these people around. So much noise. They watch me move around this room. They tell me to leave, to get some rest."

Shooting, like fire. Electricity. An image of a hammer.

"I keep telling myself, 'It did occur. It did occur.' Make myself believe. I can't."

Sizzling, peeling, knives under the skin. Sketches of a boy swimming, a cactus, a bed of ice, a splintery club, raindrops falling on a cracked desert floor. "What rain," Deirdre thought, "what rain?"

7

At that precise moment, Patrick was caught up in the better part of a dream. Having spent his youth in Birmingham, he had a deep reservoir of tragic, sometimes beautiful images of a troubled place: sweetgum trees and Spanish moss, red clay dirt that often resembled blood, acres of abandoned farms where bitter, angry cotton shrubs stretched out to a broken horizon. As a teenager, he had been sent to a school that covered miles of this kind of land. There he had known a boy named Gabriel.

Gabriel—with hair past his shoulders, eyes blue like salvation, and a voice that seemed with every syllable to echo from the peak of some mystic mountain, a guru glancing down to say:

"You think you know
everything and
nothing haunts you.
You will learn
that it is the everything you know
that ghosts your every move."

Gabriel never actually said such things; the hollows of his voice just sounded like he should. Gabriel said things like:

"You
ever
smoke
pot?"

Gabriel had no other friends, none who mattered in Patrick's eyes. And so they spent their afternoons wandering the woods, riding the raft on the lake, climbing trees. But most often they went to a near-deserted building close to the back of the campus, where a tiny darkroom stood, stocked with ancient photography supplies and a shabby cassette player. Patrick found himself here in his dream. Ravi Shankar slowly strummed as he and Gabriel moved under the old red lights, processing images of each other in the pans of chemicals circling them. Gabriel hated those chemicals. He said:

"They'll give us cancer,
man.
If I die will you?"

This question gave Patrick pause. He stood, silently watching as an image began to emerge on the paper in front of him. First he saw the eyes, so profoundly, rigorously blue. Then the rest began to come: it was Patrick's favorite picture.

The day before, Gabriel had found a window with a large, round hole in it—caused, they hoped, by a bullet—that matched the size of his head. Patrick stood on one side with his camera and Gabriel stood on the other, forcing his face into the center of the hole, and so pushing his forehead and neck against the shattering glass, which dug precipitously into his skin. Just before he began to bleed, Patrick took the picture, the sound of his camera's shutter faintly reminiscent of the gunshot they fantasized had preceded it. Gabriel said nothing, just stared at Patrick with his far-away look—the one that typically heralded one of Gabriel's soft, simple questions—as thin trails of blood began to drip down off of him to the floor. In that moment, in that one instant of standing in a relatively nondescript place doing something relatively unremarkable, Patrick felt a violent seizure in the movement of time, as if some small part of the world had suddenly decided to claim him as belonging to it.

In the dream, Patrick watched as the image etched itself into the wet piece of paper submerged in the pan. Gabriel's face is imbedded in the glass, which looks like ice, and the cracks emanating outwards from the hole look like waves of desperation, like love, circling away from him—like fire from an early spark, like tendrils off a central spore.

8

Between wakings, Patrick shifted between easy dreams, difficult hallucinations, and something deeper than sleep, an unconsciousness that had no time, no place, no presence whatsoever. Someone would later say to him:

"Did you say *coma* or *comma?*"

"That's it," he would reply. "That's it exactly. That's exactly what it was like."

What he would eventually remember of these strange states of rest, these commas, these pauses between other moments, was their profound silence. Sounds from outside would occasionally reach him—a voice, a hum, the rush of a mop—but not in the way that sounds usually do. They would simply materialize there, hidden but known to exist, stacked like linens behind a closed closet door. In fact, everything came in this way: the touch of his mother's hand on his arm, the sound of hurried footsteps, the changes in light as machines were shifted and turned; all of these presented themselves as equal parts in an ungraspable whole, just out of reach.

That fifth time that he awoke, he had the distinct sensation of his body slipping, like oil through a funnel, back into itself. This was not an unpleasant experience, and as he came into consciousness he was laughing—that particular kind of laughter that seems to bubble up from somewhere else, rising past your heart until it flushes your brain; the kind of laughter that most people believe belongs entirely to childhood, but only because they haven't laughed it themselves for so long. It was the kind of laughter that so overwhelmed him, he would not later remember it.

He had, until he woke, been embroiled in the storyline of a vicious hallucination, one that had become so terrifyingly and unflappably real to him that the Doctors and Nurses finally gave up, summoning his mother to talk him out of it. (He later wondered, if they had only realized sooner that she was a necessary player in this extended scene—not just a last-ditch effort, a relief pitcher, a way to exempt themselves from following through—how might things have turned out differently for him? But he would just as quickly remember that these professional players are there to teach, not learn; to lead, not listen. "One lick less," he would later think, "just one lick less of those desperate maneuverings, and maybe it wouldn't have been so bad.")

Deirdre's intimate knowledge of the need to be heard graced her approach. She walked slowly, like a trapper circling a feral cat, to the far side of his bed, all the while announcing herself to him:

"Patrick, it's me, it's your mother, I'm here. I sent the others away."

He kicked against the restraints, screaming, believing in his fevered state that they were lurking just outside. At this precise moment his body burned, hot and smoking oil crisping the underside of his skin. He thought they had put it there, had injected him with it, had so poisoned him with pain that it would seep out of him and infect her. He shrieked:

"You have to get out."

Ordinarily Deirdre would have had no patience for such fears—not because they were irrational, but because they were unavoidable. But standing here watching as he was lost, she was losing him, she knew. She believed the others would give up if she could not help, would shrug and walk away, perhaps slightly rattled by the theatrics of his shouts, but content in knowing there were other, easier patients who needed their care. He was right, his mother knew, they would abandon him. She leaned down to his ear, whispered:

"Where should we go? I don't know this town. You tell me." Reaching around, she began to comb his hair with her hands, a simple gesture from earlier days, when they were alone: his father at work, his brother not yet arrived, and she rocking him out of his tears, softly scratching his hair and down his back, she rocking him into herself, while everything else, all that he knew at such a newborn age, just quietly left the room. This touch, this voice, this thought that they could escape—he visibly shrank back, at once limp against the cords at his wrists and feet, at once finally serene.

"Where should we go?" she whispered again and again, asking herself as much as him, watching as he fell back into that deepest kind of sleep, falling herself into the worst kind of calm.

Interlude

Our mother inherited her resilience from our ancestors. They had been working long before they were discovered, but our mother's fore-parents weren't given a name until 1676. That must seem like so long ago. But would it matter if we had said 1976? Our family doesn't need a name.

Even so, having been named, they were able to work faster and in increasingly imaginative ways. In the old days, before you believed they were really there at all, our ancestors could take their time, toiling away in silent isolation, free as a secret to explore whatever they fancied. And in truth the name they were given in 1676 has long since faded and gone; after a while your kind got tired of it and chose another. The family name you know us by now was christened much later, in 1838—and that name was stolen from an ancient, forgotten word that had nothing to do with living things. It referred to a stick.

To say that a stick has nothing to do with living things is more than a bit misleading. What is a stick but a lost part of a living tree? And the word itself—βακτηριον, bacterion—had had a life of its own long before it was chosen for us.

Here's an example. Centuries ago, a young, embittered Egyptian king set out to build a library whose eventual loss by fire would forever be mourned. In the height of its splendor, this library housed what even then were considered ancient classics: literary, philosophical, and scientific treatises documenting centuries of human history. The young king built his collection by sending dispatches to far-away tribes, requesting translations of holy texts; by seizing and holding original copies of any documents that entered his territories by boat; and by donating literary possessions from the heavily guarded royal coffers. He was a collector, and he knew intuitively that collecting is the germ-seed of power. His library would be his throne.

One of the king's most celebrated commissions was the translation of some ancient holy books from their native Hebrew into Greek. This translation was no simple act of wordplay, but a serious and studied demonstration of the muscle of words, their ability to move and sway, their tendency to glimmer at the threshold of knowledge and imagination, in short, their willingness to act upon the stories they tell. Where previously the books had been sacred to but one embattled tribe, now their influence swept across peoples, across differences in custom and look, even across belief.

The word that would become our family name was used ten times to make the stories of those older texts legible and relevant to those who knew Greek. In each of these mentions, the word refers to an instrument of protection, not harm. The bacterion was, for example, a stick used by David (the boy who fought a giant—and won) to select the stones he would use in battle, stones that were suitably smooth: easy to grip, and quick in the air when thrown. It was also a traveler's aid, a walking stick, used in journeys and occasionally in secret rituals, in observation of the terrible need for refugees to be constantly ready to flee. And it was, too, a kind of diviner's rod, used to mark the onset of sudden, unexpected healing. (Long before Lazarus, a young mother lost her son after a sudden collapse and quick death. She sent for a prophet, who used his bacterion to touch the boy's head, to confirm he was dead, only then to revive him again.)

In any case, all these connotations were forgotten when, much later, the word was chosen for us: once you named our family in 1838, you set out to kill us. You had no idea then that to kill us would mean to kill yourselves.

PART II

9

Coming around the head of the lake, he saw the place where sand met sidewalk 100 feet away. He loved this part of his late-night runs, when he'd already finished four laps and was nearing the end of his last. Dodging the spots where the birds had been, or where dogs had left their mark, he set his sights on that rough transition and braced himself for pavement—a better surface for training, but harder to take in the joints. Easy Oakland waves slipped past the edges of the path, leaving no trace of the secrets they carelessly kept. They say that bodies were dumped from this very shore, and every year, late summer, trawlers plunged their hooks and nets into the silty bottom to catch and remove all that remained.

But no net can capture everything. He wondered what jewelry was there, and if there were rewards for finding it. He wondered who watched nervously every August, thinking that this may be the year their sin would finally be disinterred. He looked up at the building closest to him, a Victorian manse with a renovated roof, and thought he saw someone moving behind the darkened windows—a docent, a maid, a file clerk whose years working for the Historical Society housed there went unnoticed by everyone except Payroll. Who was she, he wondered, and what pleasure did she take in the details of this troubled city's past? He imagined her speaking for a fifth-grade field trip: "Oakland's redwoods were used to rebuild San Francisco after the 1906 quake. Oakland's port was the West Coast's biggest, until a corrupt mayor gave it and its proceeds to his own private firm. Oakland was once called Brooklyn, like its sister back east in New York." She would try to make these trivia meaningful to them, but they would only hear a practiced voice whose earnestness made her seem old.

Did she shrug at the end of the day? Did she insist on staying late, long after the others had left, to clean up her already-spotless desk, straightening each file, book, and box until they all lined up into a perfectly proportioned grid? Did she dream of those long-gone years, when sunbathers and punters lounged on the green? The lake had long been closed to swimming. Did she sometimes sneak down to the edge, slip off her shoe, and dip her delicately pedicured toes just beneath the surface of that water? Did she ever jump in?

He knew he had undershot the stretch of the sand when he tripped, sharply and suddenly, at the bank of the concrete walk. He had learned as a child how to fall, but—as is often the case with learning—he forgot what to do now that it mattered. First his arms flailed, seeking something to grab, and then they went for the ground, aiming to stop him before he was down. He thought he heard a whisper of a snap as his left wrist bent at an unholy angle and he slammed side-first onto the walk.

He lay for just an instant before springing up again, checking first if anyone had seen him fall. The woman behind the window had stopped moving, and seemed to be looking down at him from the second floor. He smiled and waved, a gesture of independence masked as good humor, before bending to dust himself off. A spot on his left arm stung but gave no other sign of offense. He felt his shorts, found a tear running from band to seam, and a dime-size blotch of red slowly broadening in girth—now a nickel, now a quarter, now nearly the width of an orange. He pulled back the layers of cloth to find a gash, not too deep, like what a distracted line cook might find on his hand the morning after a busy meal. He pressed hard into it while catching his breath, then checked the leak had slowed and shuffled off towards home. He glanced furtively up again to find the window empty.

Back at his four-room flat, Patrick stripped out of his clothes and started water running in the shower. While he waited the requisite five minutes for it to warm, he perched on the edge of the sink and began cleaning the wound. First peroxide then a salve, last a plaster to keep it closed. He gave it only the briefest of thoughts before looking again at his wrist, turning it in gentle circles to check its range. No sore spots, nothing broken, just a throb in the crease where arm becomes hand. But that cut near his hip, now clean and almost covered, winked open and shut as he climbed into the shower. It would leave a scar, a faint one that would only reveal itself deep in summer, when his skin had browned from the sun everywhere except there. He would forget about this cut until, days later, the plaster that had fallen off in his sleep would reappear as he laundered his sheets, sticking to the edge of a pillowcase, unrecognizable but for the stain of red in its middle part.

Wounds come in threes. One month later he would be buried deep in a back-room closet, sorting through boxes to find an old book. He would feel a sting on his left thigh, sharper than fire but duller than ice, and look down just as a spider leapt back to the ground. He would shriek and stomp, then bend to inspect what he had killed, catching sight of the tell-tale red hourglass as he wiped it up to throw it away. Two hours later he would notice the streaks on his leg, rush to a nearby clinic, and then watch as the mid-sized bump slowly grew into a massive boil, his skin gaping at the site. One month after that he would be in San Francisco, a street fair in June, and would burn the calf of his left leg on a footlight whose temperature gauge had failed. The scorch would blister and peel away, like the onionskin pages of an ancient map, revealing a network of throbbing tenderness beneath.

He would never know which of these three wounds gave the bacteria the introduction to him they needed. Gradually, in its own slow time, each of them would begin to pulse late at night, inflamed with the heat of infection—a serious-sounding word to mark the moment when bacteria arrive *en masse*. An onslaught of potions—injected, swallowed, rubbed into the skin—quickly follows, and this is when the real fight begins. For the medical world, it is a war of omnipotence; but for bacteria it is just a battle of survival. They know how to hide.

By the time they found the bacteria in a pocket near his hip, so many of them were there—he was such a hospitable host—that they began to occupy nearly every place they could fit.

10

It was an especially bright November. The fifth time he awoke, drapes covering the windows to his room were pinned back, and the glare of the sun was so complete he could not make out the lines that distinguished person from wall or ceiling from sky. "Am I outside?" he asked. "Am I at the shore?"

Everything was yellow—the figures standing around, the floors, his distant tucked-in legs, the doors. Even the air seemed to have taken on the hue of a gentler emergency, that color of caution lights, of yield signs, of crime scene tape, of the tow trucks that prowled the streets where he lived. It was a color that seemed to say, "If I'd only gotten here earlier I would be red."

Around the corner at the far side of the room, he heard a hushed conversation, his mother's familiar voice and another one, unknown:

"Somewhere near the femoral head. Sometime tomorrow."

"In his head? I thought you said it was lower."

"The *femoral* head. That's the top of his leg bone, the ball of his hip. On the left side."

"What are you going to do?"

"Send him to interventional radiology. They'll take pictures while they're digging around. It gives us a better view."

"Interventional—?"

"Like an X-ray, but better. Stronger. Real-time."

"Digging around?"

"They'll go inside the joint with small instruments to see how many pockets there are. They'll try to drain them without surgery. It's a minor procedure, but they can't put him under—just sedate him, so he'll be awake the whole time."

"Will he feel it?"

"They'll deaden the area topically. It won't be comfortable, but he won't feel pain."

His mother's voice intensified. "I don't understand. If he isn't comfortable, doesn't that mean he's in pain?"

A pause, a rustle of heavy fabric, a serious sigh. "Ma'am, your son has been in and out of excruciating pain for a long time now. You know that as well as anyone. This won't compare to what he's been feeling. It might not even register." Patrick could taste the impatience in the man's voice, like over-salted fish. "Look, there isn't much more I can tell you. We'll know more after the procedure."

"And what do I do in the meantime?"

"You should get some rest. We're over the hump, but we've still got a long way to go. You've been here every night since he was admitted. We've let you stay long past visiting hours, and I hear you slept in his room again last night. That's highly unusual on this floor. You should go home, prepare yourself for the days ahead."

"Home? I live on the east coast."

"There's a hotel down the street. You could get a room."

His mother let this pass. "What about his friends? They've been waiting to see him for days. Can they come in?"

"Not yet, but soon. Two at a time. Short visits. And remember he's quarantined. Everyone scrubs their hands and arms before and after. Everyone wears the robes and gloves. They can't touch him. No flowers or gifts. They should probably stand at least a few feet away."

"Where can we get extra robes?"

"Ask the nurse. One more thing. We need to do a transfusion. Six units at least. I'll stop by again later if I can. Goodnight, Deirdre."

Patrick wondered what intimacy had grown between this man and his mother that now permitted him to call her *Deirdre*. He wondered if she was similarly allowed to call him John or Barry or Mike.

"Goodnight, Doctor Phelps." The intimacy of strangers.

11

The intimacy of strangers—like riding a bus, or standing in line, or waiting out a storm under a highway overpass. People tend to huddle together when it matters most, organize themselves into discrete hierarchies of value, fall back on models of parent-and-child. Sometimes.

Other times huddling looks like chaos, with no one in charge. Several hours had passed since he had awoken, and now he was looking in what he believed to be his mother's general direction. She was sitting by the window, listening with such exquisite patience to his questions, with such honest readiness for her own unknowing replies.

"Why can't I see you?" he asked.

"You're blind right now."

"But I can see some things. I can see the wall. I can see my hand, if I hold it like this."

"I guess that's what some blindnesses mean."

"I can see the bed. I can see the light. I know that the television is on but the sound is off. Why can't I see you?"

"Your vision is lost."

He imagined his vision as a distinctly coherent body wandering the rooms of a vacant house, trying to find a window or door. "Where?" he asked, "Where is it lost?" He smiled at her, knowing she'd smile too.

"They're trying to find it," she laughed. "Like that time—"

"Like that time when I was six. Dad took me shopping and lost me. I used to follow him around with my hand in his back pocket. I remember."

"Your father," she said. "He was never good with things like that. He called me from the store, told me he couldn't find you. He wanted to know what he should do—call the police? But I knew you'd find him first. I told him to wait in one place, wait for you to see him."

"I was in the parking lot with my hand in some other's man's pocket before I realized. He looked down at me, called me 'Son.' He said, 'Son, do I know you?'"

Deirdre laughed—a little nervously, Patrick thought.

"Oh, stop it, mom. I know what you're thinking. That's not where it started. I was six!"

She laughed harder, and he imagined her blushing, doubled over from laughing. "You're just like your grandmother," she said with a smirk. "Wicked."

Sheila Bass, who had just come on shift after a long day with her grandchildren, blew into the room with all the grace of a truck driver. "Well, well, well," she said as if to a sold-out crowd, "I heard someone had finally come to. You've been a real trouble-maker, young man."

"I only *look* young. But don't tell my admirers," Patrick said.

"Huh. What admirers? You've got every other nurse on this floor threatening to quit. I'm the only one could handle you."

"Oh—God. I'm so sorry. I'm usually—"

"Zip it. They gave me overtime."

Deirdre turned. "Patrick, this is Sheila. She's been your nurse for the last few days. And she's not lying. One guy actually *did* quit."

"Over me?"

Sheila glanced down at him without tilting her head. "Don't even ask what you did." She reached to pull a cart closer, looked down at his chart. "But don't you worry about him. Chuck was his name. Nobody liked him. Always complaining about the bed pans."

"The bed pans. I don't blame him."

"Looks here," Sheila said, moving on, "like you're getting some blood tonight. Six units. How're you feeling now?"

"Compared to what?"

"You feel weak? Light-headed? Hungry?"

"All of those."

"Pain?"

"It's OK."

"One to ten. How bad?"

"I don't know. Four."

"Anything itch?"

"My back."

"We'll sit you up, maybe see if you can walk. You haven't moved in a while. Can you see?"

Silence, then a soft rush of action as his mother shifted in her chair, dropped a book, and bent to pick it up.

"We were just talking about that. I can see some things. I can't really see you."

She paused for a moment, then leaned close to his face. "Here's what you need to know. I'm big—real big. And strong. So don't get any ideas. I'm also gorgeous. If you get any ideas there, we can talk about it." He smiled, felt her hand move across his forehead. "I'm gonna do my best with you, Patrick. I promise you that. But I need you to do your best for me. No more screaming. Just tell me what you want, I'll get it. Deal?"

"Deal. Was I really screaming?"

"Like the Devil himself. We only have two beds to a nurse on this floor, so I'm half yours. Won't be that way forever. They're already talking about moving you down to the infectious disease ward."

"That doesn't sound good."

"It's a step up from here. Now you rest. I'll be back in a few minutes with your blood."

"She's a piece of work," Patrick said once she'd left the room.

Deirdre smiled. "She saved your life. I know it." She stood and walked to his bed. "She also reminds me of your grandmother."

"God help us."

"God help *me*."

Twenty minutes later Sheila was back with someone else, a timid-sounding man who shuffled when he walked and never made eye contact with anyone. She carried six bags of blood, reading from one of their labels. "Type A-Negative. Donor 653-RM-44210-A2."

He read from a form, a nasal echo to his tone: "A-Negative. 653-RM-44210-A2. Check."

"Type A-Negative. Donor 566-RJ-94372-A2."

"A-Negative. 566-RJ-94372-A2. Check."

This exchange continued until they had gone through all six bags, hanging each on a pole as they went. The man wordlessly left the room and Sheila busied herself with tubes, mumbling:

"We tried to give you one of these before. You probably don't remember. You tore out the IV, blood everywhere, a real mess."

"What does it feel like?" he asked.

"What does what feel like?"

"Transfusion."

She turned to look at him. "You believe in ghosts?"

"Are you serious?"

"*Do you believe in ghosts?*"

"No. Not really. Not ghosts."

"Then I don't know how to explain."

She twisted the end of one of the tubes away from the one leading into his arm, then plugged it into the end of the first bag.

"You may start to feel a little cold. We warmed this up some, but if you get the chills, say so and I'll get blankets."

He could faintly see a red line form and move slowly down the tube. As it grew closer to his arm, he began to feel nervous anticipation, like in the moments before sex when desire collapses into physical hunger but glistens too with humility—laying oneself open to the touch of another. Just before it entered him, as the shrinking emptiness between that blood and his arm began to disappear, he felt a rush of fear, his breath gone, his skin fevered and trembling. He knew suddenly that it was inside, could feel it first coursing up to his heart, then dispersed—everywhere. He remembered running. He remembered falling.

12

As he lay there, filled up with strangers, he wondered who would miss him first. The clerk who sold him beer once a week in the corner store. The woman who walked past him each morning with her dog, stopping to smoke a forbidden cigarette a block down the street. The dry cleaner, mechanic, gas station attendant. He wondered who thought of him—the teacher who, every year, hears the closing line of his junior-year term paper, not because it was elegantly phrased, but because of the metaphor that dangled in a particularly odd way. The man in prison who said the name Dewars more than any other proper noun, mourning that "one for the road" he drank in 1982 and all that it caused. The woman who sat next to him in the coffee shop last month and noticed that he had her dead father's eyes. He wondered how it could be that he figured more prominently, if only by accident, in the mental lives of these otherwise forgotten acquaintances, simply because he had happened to be there, to intersect for an instant in the paths their lives took. These are the contents of a life, he thought—all these crossings that carve out a place in the world in such unremarkable ways.

Hours after the transfusion, having struggled to think through every step that he took in an ordinary day, Patrick was flushed with the presence of those he did not know. He was surrounded by them, the faces and figures of women and men whose names he'd never heard but who were nonetheless more regular, more common to him than anyone he would have claimed as family, lover, or friend. And then there were the other others, the new strangers, who were now there, too, mixing within him like a well-rehearsed coup.

"A cocktail party," he murmured.

"A what?" Deirdre asked.

"It's like a cocktail party. Not like ghosts."

Deirdre thought he was dreaming—one of many times in the months to come when something he said would send her running to the nurses, "He's hallucinating again. Come quick."

"This blood. It's like a cocktail party. My veins the bar."

Deirdre watched as his eyes, unseeing, fluttered back-and-forth between her and the door. He seemed to have filled out in the short time since the drip had ceased, his skin now again the color of someone alive. She noticed, as she first had several decades ago, how his features mirrored those of the women in her family—her own, her sisters', his grandmother's. No one ever thought he was his father's son, so completely did he resemble her, as if her genes had by sheer force of will split apart, half of them slowly becoming him. She had worried that she carried her grief so deeply within her cells that it would be his too, and that he would eventually find himself, nearing sixty, completely infused with a will to be alone that would never reveal itself even to those he loved. He would have mystified them with his charms, she thought, so that his inevitable withdrawals would forever seem, for lack of better words, unlike him. She herself had long ago closed, like a flower—like a flower at daybreak despising the sun.

"Like a flower," Deirdre muttered as she again stroked his hair, thinking of the foul taste that word left on her tongue.

Patrick thought, as children often do, that his mother was talking about him. He turned his eyes to where he thought she was, said, "I'm too old to be a flower. Call me something else—maybe a handsome rock, a weathered seashell, a beautiful petrified tree." He smiled.

He was none of those things, she thought, but no matter. "OK. You're a tree."

13

That night he dreamed of molecules and other tiny things, of how they shift and change in the flow when matter assumes new shapes. He saw, as he slept, a drop of water down to its bones—the hydrogen and oxygen bits and all their constituent parts, floating together and apart again as the drop fell flatly to the ground. He murmured aloud, "I don't get molecules, or the spaces between."

Patrick's father Jonathan, who had arrived to relieve Deirdre of her late-night supervision, was sitting stock still in a chair across the room. He had been unable to move or sleep for the hours since he'd come, staring without ceasing, but humming along to a song about Calvary that played in his head. When Patrick spoke—for the first time since falling asleep—Jonathan stood swiftly and moved over to the bed. "What is it, son?"

Patrick's eyes fluttered open. "I don't understand molecules."

Jonathan was not a scientist, had never been into a lab, and did not know what, precisely, a molecule even was. "What don't you understand?"

"All that space. How do they hold together?"

Jonathan grasped the bars of the bed, rolling them forward and back across his palms. "Mm. Mm-hm."

"Like water. If you take a bucket of water, and pour other things into it, when does it stop being water and start being something else? Or does it stay water, but with something within it, flowing between its little bits?"

"Let me get the nurse."

"I don't feel myself."

"I'll get the nurse."

Jonathan turned and walked to the door. As he reached for the knob, Patrick said:

"Where are all of the chairs?"

"The chairs?"

"Yes, the chairs. They were just here. So small, like place-markers for a game. They were just here."

Jonathan felt a chill. "Son, what chairs?"

"Dad."

Jonathan walked partway back to the bed. "I'm right here."

"Dad, I think I had another dream, inside the first one. Or something. There were chairs, tiny, arranged all over the floor. But not here. We were someplace else, a warehouse, something like a warehouse, so big you couldn't see the walls."

"A warehouse."

"And there were chairs, arranged in long columns and rows. Perfectly spaced. Like a grid. A grid of tiny chairs. And then it changed."

Jonathan was getting invested, caught up in the scene. "How did it change?"

"Slowly, so slowly, they grew, they became huge, so you couldn't even see over them. Still in rows, still spaced apart, but bigger. I watched them grow. They were immense. They surrounded me."

"They grew ..."

"Maybe the chairs weren't changing at all, now that I think of it. Maybe it was the space that was changing. The space between. Maybe the space between, me caught in the midst of it, grew and shrank, and the chairs stayed the same. I don't know."

"The chairs stayed the same."

"I don't know, Dad. It scared me. I was scared. They kept seeming bigger, so huge you couldn't climb over them, then small again, like you would crush them if you moved."

"Like Alice. In the house. In Wonderland."

"I was so afraid."

Jonathan was now lost in his own dream-like state, swollen with thoughts of shape-shifting things. He eyes lost focus; he watched the middle-distance. "The size of things. That can be scary."

"Dad."

"Did I ever tell you about the barn behind our house? When I was a boy."

"No, I don't think so."

"I remember it being so huge. I would get lost in it. There was a top level, a loft. Loaded with hay. I don't know why there was hay up there, but it was always full of the stuff. Made me sneeze."

"Sounds like a story."

"It was horrible. My brothers would bury me in it, cover my face and the rest of me with it. I never fought back. Just lay there. Listened for them to be gone. Tried to dig myself out, it was tough with all that hay. There were things living in it. Soft rustling, a chirp, never knew for sure what those things were. Birds maybe, or a rat."

"Dad."

"And when I got out, finally kicked and pulled everything off and sat up, there I was, alone in this cave of a barn, completely dark, but not silent: sounds, little sounds, coming from all over. The things living in there."

"Hey, Dad."

"One time I sat there for hours, petrified. Mother finally came to find me. That was before Daddy died."

Patrick always grew silent at the mention of his father's father. That was a terrible story, and he didn't like hearing it. He hoped Jonathan wasn't about to tell it again. He was shivering, lying there, fully awakened from the chair-dream, so cold he thought he could see his breath. He needed his father's attention.

"It was such a huge barn. Or seemed. I went back, you know, you remember Aunt Elsie? I went back for her funeral. Stopped by the old farm. Looked at the barn."

"Dad, listen …"

"And son, you wouldn't believe it. Here I'd been remembering this huge barn, big as the world. And there it was, still a barn, but nowhere near as big as I'd remembered. Normal size. For a barn."

"Dad. Hey."

"Like it changed shape. Like your chairs. Between my memory and the realness, the realness of the barn itself. It had swollen up in my head, took up space. Moved in. And there it was. Normal size barn."

"*Dad.*"

"What?" He eyes slipped back into focus; he now saw what was there in the room. On the bed, Patrick was trembling, his whole body, every part of him. Jonathan seized to attention. "*Son.* What is it? Are you OK?"

"Dad. I'm cold. I'm freezing. It's so cold in here." His teeth started to chatter, knocking against one another like dried beans in a maraca, but with a sound less hollow than that. Jonathan pulled the door open, fast, then stood at the doorway, yelled down the hall:

"Help! I need a nurse! Hey, sir, I need a nurse!"

"Dad? You don't need to yell." He could barely make words, his teeth were shaking so hard.

"*Sir.* I need a nurse. *Now.*"

Patrick could faintly hear a voice calling back. "Hey, it's 2 a.m. Give me a minute. I'll find somebody."

"I need a nurse *now.*" A beeping sound now accompanied his father's panic, measured in the upper range, *vivace* but slightly muffled.

"Listen, calm down. Hey, Bea …" The voices trailed away.

He had slipped, or was slipping, as if through a tunnel buried deep in the floor. He could see the room from his hospital bed; it grew smaller, as through a peephole when backing away. Before he was gone, he thought: "Just like the chairs. Must have been an omen. It's all getting smaller now, like a miniature room, through a glass. It will return."

"It will return …" he started to say, but wasn't sure it all came out. In his last sight of the room, a rush of activity, someone new craned over him, peering down, then a look of shock, a turn away, a hand pulling something up and close to his neck, and then a giant whoosh as the scene, now tiny and sharp, snapped suddenly down and away.

14

It's odd, what darkness can do. As soon as the room and everything in it was gone, he found himself in a place—it was a distinct place, he felt—with no light, no windows or doors, or none he could see or otherwise sense. It was a place both with and without dimension, a peculiar quality of both being-there and being-nowhere-at-all that implied the "there" didn't matter, or wouldn't materialize, or didn't care. There are many kinds of darkness, of course: some empty, others with content so rich it can take small forevers to work it all out; some cold, others with a uniform warmth that feels like home; some solitary, others filled up with nearly-suffocating company. This particular darkness was bounded and fixed, timeless but temporary, comfortable but unrecognizable. It did not seem anonymous, but he knew he was alone. It was not silent, but this did not mean that there was sound: it was as if silence was a thing, an object, a body, that just happened not to be in this place. He could feel the existence of, but could not exactly hear, an epileptic clatter, a symphony of panic, that incessant tonal blare. He was aware that here, too, was the sensation of hands rubbing his arms and legs frantically. But he could not feel them in the usual way, perhaps because this particular darkness was not one in which he was (or was *in*) his body. But he knew they existed, the hands, the arms and legs, the friction of being rubbed.

How strange, how mystical, how Kabbalistic, this all must sound. How *New Age*. It is not as if he was *actually* outside his body, not in the way you might be imagining; but, rather, as if his body had decided to protect him from the experience that was happening to it, to remove him from the scene in the only way it knew how: by shutting down and closing up those bodily ways of knowing that mediate between us and the world outside. In a word, it simply *withdrew* him, pulled him deeper within itself, wrapped him up in its own protective, impenetrable cocoon. And there he was, excused from the business of witnessing this most recent catastrophe, this most recent collapse.

It was a darkness in which *duration* had no meaning and no effect. But there were several points—we cannot say "times" or "moments"—at which he toggled back to the room, as if it were a warped slide that just needed the right carousel slot in a projector. It would snap into place, all of it: nurses grouped over him, reaching down to him, trying to warm him up; the strange light of the hospital at night, sharp and cold and uneven, unflattering in the extreme; his father standing back in a corner, arms flanking his sides, eyes huge like moons; and the smell, that smell, meant to indicate robust sterility but stinking instead of death—sweet, too sweet. He felt no attachment to that place, nor to the comforting darkness, and experienced the toggling back-and-forth as if it were a tug-of-war between teams he was not on. And when he was fully back, wrapped now in what felt like a dozen fleece blankets with a heating pad balanced preciously on top, he felt for the first time a panic that something devastating had almost happened but had narrowly been deferred. A tall, muscular man consulted privately with his father. He heard: "We call them the death shakes around here." The man caught a glimpse of Patrick's eyes, now open and watching in his direction. He turned away from Jonathan and walked straight to the bed.

"Patrick. Welcome back. Are you warming up?"

"Hi. I, I think so. I'm warm. Actually I'm hot. Can you take this thing off?"

"No, Patrick, not yet. It's a warming blanket. We need to keep your temperature up. It's good that you feel hot, Patrick. Better than cold."

"OK. What's happening? What happened?"

"We just had a little scare, Patrick. Can you hear me OK? Can you see me, Patrick?"

"Yes, mostly. Can you stop saying my name so much?"

The man smiled and sighed a gentle laugh. "Yes, I can. I just want to make sure you stay awake. Which, clearly, you are."

"What *was* that?"

"Why don't you tell me? What did you feel?"

"Wait, who *are* you?"

"I'm Aamir. I'm one of the nurses on this ward. We haven't met, but I've heard a lot about you."

"Oh God. Do I need to apologize to you, too?"

Aamir laughed again, sweetly, compassionately. "No. And by the way, you don't need to apologize to anybody." Patrick watched him carefully, delicately: this tall, laughing man had positioned his face exactly in the spot where Patrick could see him, could make out his eyes, could appreciate his considerable beauty. Aamir knew him better than he would admit, Patrick thought.

"That's nice to hear, but I don't believe you. Apparently I've been difficult."

"Forget all that. Tell me what you felt just now." His eyes did not waver from Patrick's; his hand pressed urgently, almost lovingly, on Patrick's arm.

"Hard to explain. I had a weird dream, like a nightmare but more real. Things were changing size, proportions out of whack. Then I was talking to Dad. He was telling me a story about a barn. I kept getting colder, couldn't get warm."

"And then what?"

"My teeth were rattling, and then I was shaking. Out of control. Couldn't keep still. Kept trying to tense myself up to stop it. That didn't work. I was freezing. That's when Dad called you, I guess."

"Yes. What happened next?"

"I don't know how to describe it. Everything happened so fast, but it all kept getting smaller. Then it was gone, like it was a movie all along and someone just turned off the lamp."

"Mm."

"And then, I don't know, everything was dark. I knew things were happening, I knew people were here, but that's all I could do: *know* they were here."

He had started to sweat, drenching the blankets. He felt slightly nauseated, as if he were peering down the side of a building from its top floor. He closed his eyes.

"Patrick. Please, don't go to sleep yet." Aamir squeezed his arm then ran his hand down to Patrick's own, laced his fingers, held them. "I can't let you go to sleep yet. Stay with me, OK?"

"OK. I'm here. That was so … well, weird."

"Are you thirsty? Hungry? Do you want something to eat?"

"I liked that pistachio pudding earlier. I like strawberry milk."

Aamir laughed again. "Jonathan, will you please walk down the hall to the nurses' station? Tell Bea that I need some of the green pudding and some strawberry milk. She'll call down to the kitchen. And then please go downstairs and take a few minutes outside, OK? Look at the stars. Stretch your legs. I need to talk to Patrick privately."

"OK." Jonathan was very good—always had been—at being told what to do. "I love you, son." He turned and left, willing himself to breathe, willing himself to walk, willing himself to forgive himself for never knowing on his own what he should do.

15

"Have you been tested?"

Alone now in the room, Aamir leaned over Patrick, still holding his hand, and gazed expectantly down at him. Patrick shifted uncomfortably under the blankets and pad, tried to adjust his legs. He took a deep breath, turned to look at the door, then looked back towards Aamir.

"Have you been tested?" Aamir asked again.

"It's funny how that question works," Patrick said. "Used to be like 'Hello,' in certain places I mean. At certain times. 'Have you been tested? Oh, and I'm Patrick, by the way.' Waiting for an answer to know what would happen next. You know what I mean."

"Yes," Aamir said, "I do. So much tension built up in it. So much possibility. But so much fear, too."

"I remember the first time I asked it. It was such an *event*. Something I'd had to learn how to do. I was in college, in Chicago, standing by the lake, and I was so nervous. 'Have you been tested?' I asked, and he turned and laughed at me. 'Are you kidding? Of course I have. Every month.' Every month! I couldn't believe it. 'That's too much,' I said. 'You'll drive yourself crazy.' 'I have a lot of sex,' he said. 'Still. Still,' I said, 'too much.'"

Aamir smiled. He raised an eyebrow, smirked, said: "So, Patrick, have you been tested?" He smiled again, broader this time, cheeky.

Patrick laughed. "Yes. Every six months. Last time was two months ago—or three. I don't know, I've lost track of time. It was in August I think."

"So you're sexually active?"

"Not at the moment. Unless holding hands counts."

Aamir smiled again, squeezed Patrick's fingers. "Do you know your risk factors?"

"Why are you asking me these things? I mean, why now?"

"Well, your father was supposed to ask you about this. I mean, not these questions exactly; he was supposed to ask you about having a blood test. We can't just do it without asking. You have to consent, go through the interview first."

"Oh. Right."

"But between you and me, I don't think your father's ready for that conversation."

"I don't think he's ready for any of this."

"No. But this might just push it over the top. So, listen. They want to test you. Not the standard—for antibodies—but the viral DNA test. Just to make sure."

"Make sure I'm not positive?"

"Yes. They found the bacteria, they believe that's the cause. They just want to make sure there's nothing else." Aamir watched Patrick, waiting. Patrick sighed, resigned.

"Yeah. OK. That's fine." He sighed again, looked at the walls. "Gets old, you know."

"I do."

"Walk into a clinic, something's wrong, maybe a cold, a sprained ankle, a cut from a kitchen knife, whatever. 'Have you been tested?' Like it's only a matter of time. Like this might be the one. Like finally they'll get the result they expect. Inevitable."

"Yes."

"Gets old."

"It does."

"Sets up a pattern, you know? Where you start to expect it yourself. Get a sneeze or sore throat, it's the first thing you think of. Makes you wonder whether you might as well go ahead and convert, just to get it over with."

"Well. I've never heard it put *that* way before."

"I don't know. I guess it's better than not testing at all. At least there's that."

"There is that." Somewhere near the window, a fluorescent bulb flickered and faded, then popped back to life.

"You know the worst part?" Patrick asked.

"What's that?"

"When the test comes back negative, which I'm pretty sure it will, some of my family will celebrate. No matter how sick I still am. They'll celebrate. They'll tell everyone. 'Well, he's sick, sure, but he doesn't have AIDS. It's not AIDS. It's something else.' Like that matters. Like this illness, whatever it is, is somehow more wholesome, more holy, more clean, because it's not HIV."

Aamir tightened his lips, looked slightly off for a moment, then looked back at Patrick, smiled again. "Yes." A moment passed. "But you know, Patrick, they aren't responsible for everything they think. You can't hold them account-able for everything. They inherit so much—*we* inherit so much—without knowing any better."

"That's generous. That's kind. And you're right. Still makes me angry. How dare they. You know? How *dare* they moralize what is happening to me. No one *deserves* to get sick. *No one.*"

"No one deserves to get sick." Aamir shook his head, back-and-forth.

They sat then for a few minutes (it could have been five or ten) in silence. Patrick wanted to close his eyes but remembered that he needed to stay awake. He liked the feeling of Aamir's hand on his, wanted to fall asleep feeling it. He thought of the spaces between his fingers, how they begged for others to fill them. He thought of standing by the lake, of that question, its answer, his own. He thought of secrets and what they tell. He thought of rain.

"When I was twenty-six," Aamir started, then stopped. Patrick looked towards him. Aamir's eyes were large and soft, his mouth slightly open, his head sunk just enough to give the impression that he was day-dreaming. Patrick waited, drifting himself into the lower registers of being-awake. Aamir sniffed, licked his lips. "When I was twenty-six, my lover died."

Despite the heightened presence its content called for, this sentence did not startle Patrick or jar him further awake. It seemed instead to lie down next to him, to join him in repose.

"He died slowly, over many months. I was an artist then. I worked in metals." Aamir briefly let go of Patrick's hand, reached up to scratch a spot on his neck, then reached down again. Patrick noticed how warm and dry his fingers felt, how thick and strong, so unlike his own.

"I was a slow worker. It took me weeks, sometimes months, to finish a single piece. It was a tortuous process. Not painful. Just long." He spoke slowly, choosing his words. "They sent him home from the hospital very early. Nothing they could do. And they needed the bed. I moved him into my studio. Set up a mattress near where I worked, but not so near that the noise would bother him. He liked to watch me, and I didn't mind.

"About two weeks in, he started making requests. 'Make me a little tree, Aamir.' Or, 'Make my mother a ring.' And I did. I always did. Once he asked for a special prong, one he could balance on his chest to hold a book open. I made that one out of silver, rimmed its base with tiny stones, etched his name along its spine. He liked it so much he refused to put it away, even when there was no book. It stayed next to him in bed." Patrick tried to imagine the shape of the silver, its sheen, the look of the stones. He did not ask what was the name drawn into it.

"And I knew, long before he asked, what he wanted me to do with it. I could tell, over time, that he was spending so much time with it so as to fill it with himself, like a charm, or a talisman. Like a relic."

"What books did he read while he was sick?" Patrick asked, unsure if he should interrupt, but too curious not to. Aamir looked up, thought.

"Wow. I don't remember. Let's see. He liked James Baldwin. *Giovanni's Room*, *Tell Me How Long the Train's Been Gone*. And Highsmith. *Cry of the Owl*. The *Ripley* series. He must have read those, or re-read them. He loved books. Loved spending time with them."

"I love Baldwin and Highsmith, too."

"I've never read her. I don't really like mysteries." Patrick let this pass.

"Did he talk about them?"

"Not really, no. Sometimes he would laugh out loud, or become sad at some little part. He'd try to explain it to me, but he wasn't good at summarizing things. He would just talk on and on, confusing himself and me. Finally he'd just give up, roll his eyes, and go back to his book. To be honest I was always slightly jealous of those books. Like I couldn't live up to the characters inside them, like I wasn't interesting enough."

"Hm."

"Yeah, 'Hm.' Silly. But jealousy always is." Aamir rocked back slightly, rolled his fingers so that they turned back-and-forth against Patrick's. "When he died, the night he died, it was cold outside, one of those intensely cold nights that fools you into thinking we live in a place with seasons."

"I love those nights."

"So do I. So did he. It was so cold, and the studio didn't have enough heat. I had moved him into the living room that day, near the fireplace. I went and bought some wood: I remember it was from an avocado tree. Those details. Strange how we remember them. Avocado wood. I remember how good he seemed, like he was somehow on a recovery. He was laughing just minutes before, laughing uncontrollably at some joke I'd told that really wasn't all that funny. Don't ask—I don't remember what it was." He paused. "Ha. Think about that. I can remember what kind of wood was burning, but I can't remember what I said the last time I made my lover laugh."

Patrick thought it wasn't really all that strange. Probably Aamir did remember, but had locked the joke away, keeping it so private that even he didn't know it was still there. He kept this thought to himself.

"He was laughing, and I went into the kitchen to make some tea. It took me too long. I boiled the kettle and rinsed out the pot, which cracked and broke when I poured the hot water in. So I had to start all over. By the time I was back by the fire, he was gone. His eyes were open, and he had what looked like a little frown on his face. But he was gone. I put down the tea, sat with him for a while. Held his hands in mine. Watched him. Waited. When I finally called the doctor, it was past midnight."

Patrick lay still, absorbing the moment. Some time passed before Aamir continued.

"Once they had taken him away, it was four in the morning I think, I noticed that he had put the little silver book holder on the floor next to the mattress I had pulled in there, next to a piece of paper. I hadn't noticed it before. I didn't even know he had paper or pencil with him. But there it was: a note in his cursive. 'Keep this. Do not bury it with me.'

"That was the first and only time I sobbed, I mean really lost it. Right there on the floor, holding this scrap of paper with his handwriting on it, wadding it up I was crying so hard. I didn't dare touch the silver prong. I could tell, even in the light from an old floor lamp, that it was covered in him, his fingerprints smeared all over it. I left it where he had put it, right there on the floor, through the wake, through the services, through the visits from friends checking up on me, making sure I was alright. I left it there as long as I could.

"And then one ordinary day, a Tuesday I think, a month or so later, I came into the room and saw it there, and I went and picked it up and put it away. Not far away, not packed in a box, just put away. Out of sight. And on that day, that very afternoon, I packed up my studio, started selling all my tools. Gave it up. Walked away. Turned the studio into a guest room. Signed up for my first nursing class. And the rest, you know …" He trailed off, then looked sharply at Patrick, smiled. "The rest pales in comparison to what came before. Not worse. Just a different life. Less vivid. Less intense."

Patrick squeezed Aamir's fingers, held them. Aamir squeezed back, quick and firm, then stretched down with his other hand to feel Patrick's forehead. He brushed the hair that lay there to the side, then placed the full length of his hand along the side of Patrick's face.

"You are tired," he said. "You should sleep. You're OK now. I'll take the warming pad away. Sleep well, Patrick. Sleep deep."

16

Deirdre sat in the chair closest to the window, watching out for the nearly-winter sun. She was an early riser, always had been. Didn't care much for sleep. A notebook lay open on her lap. In it she had written "Tuesday" and "morning" and "sleeping well," and had drawn a small circle surrounded by clouds. And then, without thinking, she had drawn two eyes and a smile inside the circle. She was waiting for morning rounds.

Jonathan had barely survived his first night staying with Patrick. Deirdre had received a phone call at 4 a.m., his soft, rolling voice more scattered and broken than usual, clearly undone. She couldn't tell if something very serious had happened or if Jonathan was over-reacting. "No matter," she had decided. "I'm awake anyway. I'll just go."

"Where's Sheila?" she had asked at the desk. "When does she come in?"

"Should be here by six."

"Who was here overnight?"

"Aamir. He sat with your son."

"I thought it was someone named Barb."

"Barb was on a break when it happened. Aamir took over. Have you met him yet?"

"No."

"He's with someone else right now. He'll probably be in to see you soon."

Deirdre did not care for imprecision. But her mother had taught her that nurses were always already-overwhelmed, and were almost always doing the best they could. So she had gone back to Patrick's room, where Jonathan stood by the bed, still looking traumatized. Patrick was asleep, a sleep so deep his presence in the room was nothing more than a technicality. She sent Jonathan back to his hotel. "Get some rest. You did well, Jonathan. Thank you. I needed a break. Thank you, really. I'll call you later, OK?"

"Do you know what time the procedure is happening?"

"I'm not sure. Probably around 10 or so. I don't know if they'll want to hold off because of what happened last night. I can call you as soon as I know."

"I'd like to be here."

"Of course. Yes, of course. I'll call you."

A moment passed between them, silent and small. They had been married for nearly twenty years before the divorce. They could not help but pass moments of unspoken intensity together from time to time. It was all of a piece.

"I'll call you."

"Thank you. For everything. You know I couldn't do what you've done."

"Jonathan, really, we are all doing everything we can. All of us. You too. Please, go get some rest. I'll call."

"OK."

"OK."

She sat, waiting for the deep blackness of the night to begin its slide into dark royal blue. It was almost 5:30. There was a soft knock at the door, so soft it might have been a footstep. She brushed off her lap, took one last look out the window, stood, and turned.

"You must be Deirdre."

Deirdre's hand unconsciously went to fix her hair, to soften its harsh angles. She blinked several times. The man at the door was stunning. His bright green eyes seemed to travel fully across the room just to be next to her. His smile was warm and full.

"Yes. Hello." She matched his smile, or tried to. She felt the muscles of her face stretch and pull. "Are you …?"

"Aamir. Yes." He took a few steps into the room. "Is he still sleeping?"

"Yes. He hasn't woken up since I got here. He's barely moved."

"Good. Rough night."

"I heard. And you were here?"

"Yes. Your … Patrick's father called me in when it started. I stayed with him afterwards, until he fell asleep."

"Thank you."

"Of course. I was happy to be here. We talked for a while. After."

"Was he …" Deirdre finally turned to look at her son. "Was he coherent? Was he making sense?"

"Well, to be honest, I did most of the talking. But yes. He was very present, very much awake. I would say 'very much himself,' but I don't know him well enough to say that, so …"

Deirdre turned back to Aamir. "I'm sure he appreciated it. Enjoyed it. Thank you."

"Of course."

"You work with Sheila?"

"I do. She's one of the best."

"I like her. Patrick likes her, too."

"Just stay on her good side."

"Do you know if they're going to go ahead with the—"

"The radiology? I don't. I see that it's scheduled. The doctor will talk to you about it when he comes in, will make the decision then. Patrick is stable, but last night was a bump. So we'll see."

Deirdre smiled again, smaller this time, lips together.

Aamir walked to the bed, peered down at Patrick, then walked to Deirdre. "I'm off in a few minutes. I won't be in again until tomorrow night, late. Will you tell Patrick that I'll stop by to see him when I can?"

"Thank you. I will."

"Tell him I'm rooting for him."

"Thank you."

"He's lucky you're here."

"Where else would I be? *Could* I be?"

Aamir smiled. "Yes. I know. Still."

An hour or so later, Deirdre and Sheila were looking together at the charts from the night before. Sheila looked pained, as if she couldn't quite understand what Aamir had written. Deirdre was trying to follow, too, was trying to transcribe some of what Sheila was reading to her, into her notebook. They were interrupted by a group of white-coated men and a single young woman, who charged like a herd noisily into the room.

"Well, Mister Anderson," boomed the one in front, "how are we feeling today?"

Sheila turned fiercely around: "He's asleep, Doc. Rough night."

"I see that. Let's wake him up, please, um, Sheila."

Into the brief instant before she turned to the bed, Sheila packed such intense and obvious disregard for this man that Deirdre thought it might explode. But it did not. Sheila woke Patrick by holding his shoulder, gently, then squeezing it, saying, "Patrick. Patrick, I need you to wake up. The Doctors are here for morning rounds."

As it happened, the Doctor on-call had had nothing to say of any value. His charges—new residents in the hospital, fresh out of Med School—were just along for the ride, the learning, and so were of little interest or use to Deirdre. Two hours later, Doctor Phelps returned to give the go-ahead. He seemed unsurprised by the events of the previous night.

"Happens," he said to Deirdre.

"What do you mean?"

"Happens from time to time. Looks dramatic from the outside. But it usually just passes. Only two ways it can really turn out, after all. Either they're back or they're not."

Sheila glanced up, shot Deirdre a quick "don't bother" look from behind the Doctor's back, then returned to the IV, gripping Patrick's arm.

"Right. Well. What time will they take him down?"

"Same as we said. 10. Might be a bit later if they're backed up."

"Are you doing it?"

"No. I'm a hospitalist, Deirdre. Doctor Montgomery will do it. Hands are his specialty, but he's done the other joints before. He's young, but he's good. Maybe he'll stop by before."

It was a rush of a morning once Sheila had arrived. Moments after Doctor Phelps and Sheila had both left the room, an exuberant if absent-minded man who looked far too young to be a surgeon nearly tripped as he entered.

"Oopsy. Ha-ha. There we are, all steady. So … Anderson. Patrick. Patricio."

"You?" Deirdre said in greeting.

"Hello. Are you the mom?"

"Are you Doctor Montgomery?"

"Call me Monty. Please."

"You're the Doctor? The one who's doing the procedure?"

"The same."

Deirdre wished that Sheila were in the room so she would know how to feel. On one hand this man seemed human. On the other he seemed like the vice-president of a second-tier fraternity.

"So," he continued, "let's talk about what we're doing. Is ..." He shuffled through his papers again. "Is Patrick awake?"

"I am, hi."

Monty looked up. "Hi there. Woah. You look great."

"I do?"

"For what you've been through, yes. You look outrageously great. I was expecting someone who looked like he'd been in a bar fight."

"I feel like I've been in a bar fight."

"You been through much worse than that. And you. Look. Great." He pointed as these last words came out.

"Well. Thank you. You look great too."

"Ha-ha! Do I? I don't hear that too often. Gotten a little soft."

In spite of herself, Deirdre was vaguely smiling: a soft, summery smile, the kind you see on people while they're watching children on a playground, getting along. A smile without longing, without reservation, without worry.

"So," Monty went on, "let's talk." He walked to the edge of the bed, lowered the bars on that side, and sat, half-perched on the thin mattress. "Here's what's happening. You've got abscesses in your hip. All over. A few of them are quite large, bigger than we'd expect in that area. Many more are quite small. I need to get them out. That is to say, I need to drain them."

Deirdre snapped out of the smile, walked to the chair and sat down in it. She pulled out the notebook, began scribbling. "Where are they again?" she asked.

"In the left hip, near the femoral head. But scattered, too, down along the femur. There might be some further in, around the pelvis. We're not sure. That's why I need to go in and have a look-see."

Deirdre kept writing. "I hear you're good with hands," she said as she wrote.

"Yes! Hands are what I do. They're amazing, you know, hands. So intricate. Difficult. Complex. Puzzles, all of them."

"Have you ever worked on a hip?"

"Oh yes, no worries there. I've worked on hips. And ankles and knees and shoulders and even, once, on an elbow. My mentor was a hip man. I just decided to branch out."

"I see. So you're confident you can do this."

"Oh yes. Well, it's a difficult procedure. Not dangerous," he turned back to face Patrick, pointed, "*not dangerous*, I want to be clear. And you won't feel much. Shouldn't hurt, might feel a little strange. That's all. I've done one like this before. Very similar case. Well, not quite as intense. But similar. Came out very well, if I say so myself."

"Tell me," Patrick said, "what exactly are you going to do?"

"Sure, sure." He set his papers down on the bed and sketched this next part out in the air, his fingers moving with quick precision around an imagined stretch of skin. "I'll make a small incision—won't know *how* small until we're there, depends on what we find—on the front side of your left hip. We'll be running a CT scan while we do this, watching ourselves work on screen. You'll be awake, relaxed with some lorazepam but otherwise awake, and the area will be locally anesthetized. Once we get going, I'll track the abscesses, then begin draining them with very thin needles. Depending on how far we get with that, I might need to leave some small catheters in place so the drainage can continue. Depends."

"Is this really going to help?" Deirdre asked, more sharply than she intended. Monty turned to look at her, startled but unoffended. "I'm sorry. But is it?" she said.

Monty turned to look at Patrick, then back at Deirdre again. "I'm not going to blow smoke up your ass, either of you. This isn't a cure-all. But we think this is the root of the problem—these clusters, these abscesses, are where those little buggers are hanging out. Usually the immune system can handle it, can clear them away. That's not happening here, in part because the bacteria are of such a virulent strain, completely resistant to all but one or two antibiotics. So we need to remove them … well, manually, I guess, in addition to pumping you full of the right drug. It's messy; but yes, it will help."

"OK. Patrick? Honey? Any questions?"

"I don't think so. Wait. Can I watch the screen?"

Monty smiled. "I thought you might ask that. *No.* Sorry, buddy, but no."

"Why not?"

"One, because I need you to be still and relaxed, not caught up in the show. Two, because I have a feeling that you would want to be involved, telling me what you see, telling me what to do."

Patrick smiled at this. "Probably."

"So no. Sorry. Anything else?"

"How long will it take?"

"Probably a while. A few hours. Maybe more. Just depends."

"OK."

"OK. Anything else you want to ask, mademoiselle?"

Deirdre smirked. "I think I'm good. Take care of my son."

"Oh, I will. I will. You can take *that* to the bank."

"OK then."

"Alright, then, I'll see you soon, champ." And with that and a wink, he blustered out of the room.

Interlude

You might wonder: did we understand this conversation as it occurred? Did we recognize it for the threat that it was? Did we fortify ourselves in some way, preparing for the onslaught of attack? Did we begin devising a response?

We did not.

But we did hunger, feeling deep deprivation as we longed to expand and that sharp desire to return that follows an attack. We were down, but not yet dead—and we ached for a restoration of the communal well-being that we so love.

Perhaps it is difficult for you to think of us in human terms—as those who hunger, as those who love. Perhaps it is unimaginable, the notion that we might have opinions at all, much less opinions of one another, of other figures, of other beings. Perhaps you think it cannot be so; perhaps you dismiss the very idea as ridiculous, as childlike in its imagi- nation and naïveté, as myth. While it is probably true that we do not experience the realm of emotions as discrete—we have no names for them among ourselves—it could not be further from the truth that we do not undergo attraction, repulsion, closeness, rupture, in a word, desire. We are your distant kin, after all: modern-day descendants of those first fated cells that jumped with a spark from the gods and sprang to life. We are just as evolved as you. We have survived just as long—longer, in fact—battling it out to survive our environments, to model and rehearse those genetic aberrations that have given us our edge. Can desire be so far off? Is it so difficult to imagine longing as a minor deviation when compared to the triumph of enduring across inconceivable numbers of millennia?

Some among you know of our power, and treat us as seriously—as honorably—as they treat you. Some among you spend their lives tracking and telling our stories. Some take us so seriously they spend their lives attempting to eradicate us, or some of us at least, from the planet. They know, of course, that such a thing is unlikely—impossible to prove, even if they thought they'd done it. But still they try. And still they fail—so piti- fully that they jump scale, from the planet to a body, a single body. Imagine that: they set out to kill us off and then, realizing their farce, find ways simply to banish us from a single human body, one at a time. Soaps, wipes, medicines, materials, so many developed just to keep us at bay. From a single site or soul. One at a time.

The irony, of course, is that in order to develop these strategies, they first must nurture great numbers of us in their labs. They must seduce us to thrive and expand, to reproduce our numbers, to sustain ourselves in those tiny, constricted glass homes. They bring us up, feeding us, strengthening us, building up our resources, and then switch to see what will work to shut us down, quick as you like. You have no idea how many failures this process has entailed. So few things work, and looking and trying take time.

In the early days you began, as you so often do, by trying to see us, as if visibility were the key to existence. What you call the Enlightenment was defined by that will to see, on both large and small frontiers: the cosmos alongside the minutiae in a wild, rowdy obliteration of the barriers of scale. You discovered bent, rounded glass as a mediator, a shaper of light that could bring into focal relief what was otherwise only hypothetical. Armed with such an implement, in the seventeenth century, a Dutch draper from Delft discovered that in most substances there exist tiny worlds of what he called "nimble creatures," organisms that had evaded your notice until positioned beneath the glaring point of his specialized device, raised and lowered to capture differing layers of depth.

He had first aimed this odd tool at rain water, collected in a small clay pot, and found there hundreds of swimming beasts, hedging into or scattering away from the center of the image. He looked up and backed away, rubbing his eyes, opening and closing them several times, then peered into it again. And there they were, still swimming, a world of complexity where few had expected (and none had seen) it before. He watched their tails propel them forward and back again, sometimes becoming stuck on a tiny piece of dust or thread. Their bodies would then turn around, seeking the end of the tail, suffering there with frantic windings and quiverings to disentangle themselves from the trap.

He collected more rain, each day closer to the source: next straightaway from the gutter, gathering it up in a bowl; then in a heavily-washed glass, direct from the sky. Even there, even thus, he found some like us, in the purest of cloudburst samples, smaller and fewer, more pellucid, harder to find, but still there. It was a remarkable discovery: like a bee to a horse, he wrote in an attempt to fathom their relative size, so these poor little creatures are to the eye of a mite.

Not trusting his own expertise, the man wrote to the Royal Society—then the chief collector of such observations—to describe what he saw: long, flowing letters, lush with detail about both the creatures and his exercises at finding them. He could not summon the sense of self-worth to gather together a proper case study, not seeking fame—so he simply wrote letters, hundreds of them, describing what he saw, and how, and when, and what had been happening while he looked. They were thick with narration, his missives, exuberant in the delight of looking, but not with the ostentation of one who is the first to see: they were humble, a rare form for the Society, one it was not quite sure how to handle. He wrote even from his deathbed, now ninety—a ripe age for the time—to say that he had spied us again in the muscles and sinews of large, already-classified beasts. We were everywhere, in everything, populating the living and unliving stuff of the world, beings that had infiltrated all but the coldest and hottest of Earth's materials.

It was not long before you connected the dots and began blaming us—not just our family, but all of us, there on the microscope's plate—for an ever-increasing range of illnesses that plagued your kind. For 100 years before the young Dutchman's revelation, there had been sacrilegious whispers about what some called germs, the unseen ontologies of contagion and disease. And within 100 years of his death, others had found means to prove the link. A great cascade of discoveries, then, about our passage from one host to another, our varying effects upon your systems, our sometimes-relationship to imminent decline.

How can you not see desire at play in our work—at the very least, a desire to survive? We may be just as evolved as you, and older; but this does not make us any less vulnerable, any less susceptible to the inevitable, any less affected by yearning and any less eager to yield to its calls. We yearned to remain, as we ceaselessly do—and we are still here.

PART III

17

Patrick was slowly waking up. Not in the immediate sense, of coming out of a nap; but in the more profound way: he was slowly coming to understand the length and breadth of what had happened, of what was happening. Where in the previous weeks his understanding was fractured and temporary at best, limited to what was right before him, or had only just passed—limited, too, by the sense of things his dreams and hallucinations left in their wake—now he was beginning to piece longer periods of time together, to comprehend the broad outlines (though not yet the specifics) of our shared story's beginnings, to comprehend that he currently occupied its middle. As awakenings of this sort are wont to do, this one also began to nurture in Patrick a longing for the story's end, a desire to know how things were shaping up and when things would begin to take their place as part of his past.

This slow awakening did not yet manifest itself as impatience, but rather as curiosity: he grew more involved in his own care. Not yet strong (or, indeed, awake) enough to shoulder it all, he still looked to Deirdre to collect data, to ensure the right questions were asked, to help him make decisions when prompted about whether or not to proceed with this or that course. But—much like a child advancing through grammar school, slowly coming into her own—he was more and more aware of his own subjectivity, his own person-hood, his own there-ness in the room. And he was more and more aware of us, lurking in the background of his consciousness, waiting—for nothing in particular, but waiting nonetheless.

As they wheeled his bed down the halls, into the elevator and out again, into a dark, cavernous space spotted with monstrous machines, Patrick did not think.

He focused instead on the feel of hospital air moving across his skin, on the thin flannel draped across his chest, on the tight point in his arm where the IV needle went in. It might have been a long journey or a short one; Patrick neither knew nor was aware that he didn't know. Already the lorazepam was kicking in. It was not unpleasant.

The man pushing his bed seemed to disappear, replaced by a woman with long, dark hair tied up in a bun. The bottom two-thirds of her face were covered with a white mask; her eyes were neither kind nor unkind. She said so softly he wondered if she really spoke: "Patrick, right? We're going to move you over to this platform here." She gestured to her right. Someone strong reached under his shoulders, pulled him up and over. The woman lifted from his knees, and as she pulled, a shot of righteous, physical anger shot forth from his left leg, straight up to his spine, from there to his neck, then back again, doubling down on its insistence. He was too stunned, too shocked by the jolt, to make a sound. It felt dry and solid, electric in its intensity and in the way it maintained a steady connection—a vibrating current—as it moved from hip to head. They lay him down again, this surface harder than the bed.

"Oh my God," he finally said, nearly breathless. "Oh my God, oh my God, oh my God, what is that?"

"Patrick? Something wrong?" the woman asked, moving around to his side.

"Am I in pain?" he asked strangely. "Am I in pain? Is that what this is?"

"There might be some pain," she said.

"Oh my *God*," he said.

She placed her hands palms-down on his chest. "Breathe, Patrick. Breathe slowly. I'll breathe with you. In, all the way in ..." She inhaled in a measured way, held her breath. "Now out, slowly pushing it out." A soft hissing noise, like a punctured balloon, as she breathed. "OK? Breathe again. In and out. Deep as you can."

He followed her breaths, pulling and pushing the air like a wagon of wood. It was heavy but clean, tidy and cold. He breathed. His body began to relax into itself, to release the jolt trapped there as if from a cage. "Oh my God," he said, softer now.

"Better?" she asked.

"Yes," he said. "Better."

"Good. My name is Rosario. I'm the nurse down here. I'll be assisting Doctor Montgomery. I'll be with you the whole time, right here next to you."

"Hi, Rosario. Thank you."

"It's my job," she said simply, not unkindly: a statement of fact. "I need to get a few things ready. You just keep breathing, OK? I'll be back in just a moment."

"Right. OK."

When she returned he had recovered and lay limp, looking around. Above and around to his left craned one of the massive machines, a dull claw of a shape. He could see that there was a monitor above him, but could not see its face. There were wires and tools spread out on rolling steel tables nearby. He got the gist of it all, understood how the pieces fit together and made a whole.

"I'm going to give you some more lorazepam and increase your pain meds," Rosario said. "You'll feel them." A soft rustling of cloth, a short tapping, then: "I'm pushing them in now." He could feel the cool liquid as it entered through the IV port. A flash of total bliss, complete in its perfect haziness; and then it seemed to settle, to spread over and within him, to spread him out within itself. "Yes?" Rosario asked.

"Oh—oh, yes," he said, slurring the words just a bit. "Yes, I can feel them. I can feel them just fine. Just fine now."

He became aware of a strange tugging feeling at his hip. He started to lift his head and look down at it, but was stopped by Doctor Montgomery, who held small tools that seemed to be pointed into his body, that seemed to be sticking out of his body.

"Stay still, Patrick, please."

"When did *you* get here?" Patrick asked.

"We're about thirty minutes in. Stay still, OK? Try to relax. Rosario, help?"

She walked around him and stood behind where Patrick's head lay. She placed a hand on each of his shoulders, pressed gently into them.

Patrick thought he saw an oak tree growing in the corner of the room, dropping its leaves. He wanted to get closer to it, to trace the patterns its bark held. He was about to lean in when he heard: "I can't. I can't get to them. *Jesus*, there are a lot." A heavy, snorted sigh.

He tipped his head up; "Is everything OK?" he asked the room.

Doctor Montgomery leaned in, looked down at Patrick's hip, then looked up at the screen. "We're nearly done, Patrick. Just lie still."

"Wow, that was fast."

"No, you've just been in and out. It's been about four hours."

"No way," Patrick said.

"Four hours. Not much longer. Hold tight, champ. Hold tight." The tree was gone, replaced again by the room, the machines and the shadows they cast. Something moved across his field of vision, blocked the shadows, then moved away.

Now he was rolling—no, drifting, like on a boat. Not at sea. Through a strange cave, with even white walls. No, a room—a hall. He wasn't sure, but he was moving. Someone was whistling. He popped his head back, upside down on its crown, to look behind him.

"Woah! Hi there. You back in the real world?"

"Woah," Patrick said, "woah."

"You were tripping, boy. Tripping out."

"Wo-o-oah—"

"Yeah, welcome back. Welcome back, welcome back. Welcome back to the world. Almost there, hang on." The bed cocked and wheeled to the left, turning a corner to another hall, then slowed, turned, and backed into the room.

"Here we are. Home at last, home at last."

The man steadied the bed, locked its wheels in place, plugged it back into the wall.

"Woah," Patrick said, "here we are."

"Yep. Here we are. Nurse'll be back in a minute. Take it easy." The man turned and left the room.

"OK," Patrick said. "I will." He closed his eyes, tried to place himself in time. It seemed to be dark outside, or getting there. The lamp on the table was on, soft and warm. Everything was still. "Take it easy," he said to the empty room.

He turned to the lamp. Beneath it, he saw a small ornamental tree, pewter perhaps, stretched up and out like a maple, well-pruned. It had 100 branches, or seemed to, each an intricate arm reached up towards the light. Beside the tree was a note with orderly, if ornate, scrawl: "Heal up, Patrick. –Aamir."

"He dropped by to leave that for you an hour ago," Sheila said, suddenly in the room. "On his *night off*."

"It's beautiful."

"Very talented, that one. More ways than one."

"Where is everyone?" Patrick asked. "Mom, Dad?"

"They're talking in the waiting room. They'll be back in a minute. How do you feel?"

"Loopy."

"Rosie said you were acting out."

"Was I?"

"Talking nonsense."

"How did it go? The procedure? Did they get everything?"

"Not sure. Doc Monty'll come talk to you. Hungry?"

"Starving."

"Good. It's pot pie tonight."

"I *love* pot pie."

"Lie back. I need to go check on a few things. Be back before you know it." Sheila seemed distracted, or tired. She was gone before he had decided what to say. He reached for the tree, lifted it from its perch on the table. It was surprisingly light—clearly solid, but fragile. As he drew it closer, he saw that it had been made without leaves except in one place: at the end of a branch, not the topmost branch but one not too far below, was a single tiny leaf hanging on by the most delicate of stems. The leaf was made with intense detail, pocks and veins just visible on both sides. It curled slightly at its edges, dehydrated, nearly dead: early winter, all the rest gone, this was the last leaf to hold on before dropping. The last leaf—frozen forever in place, trapped or held on its branch like a relentless recurrent dream.

18

Deirdre was writing, Jonathan and Sheila were watching, as Monty sat, disheveled, on Patrick's bed.

"I couldn't get to everything. There were so many, so many more than we'd thought. I got the biggest ones, drained them right up, and about a dozen of the small ones. But there were so many of them, scattered all over the place. Really, champ, I don't know *how* you're still alive." He pointed at Patrick's chest, pressed his finger into it. "You are a *fighter*."

"So what does this mean?" asked Deirdre, eyes fixed firm on her book. "What do we do now?"

"I mean it," said Monty, still pressing, "a *fighter*. You should be *dead*."

Patrick wasn't sure what he was supposed to feel about this: pride? He did not feel pride.

Monty craned his neck to look at Deirdre. "Not much more we can do from the inside, not at this point. We could open him up all the way, go through again, see if we can get them all. But with this kind of infection, it's too risky. If one of those things were to burst while he was open … well. Bacteria everywhere. A real mess. Big trouble."

"So you're just going to leave them there?"

"Yes. For now. The infectious disease people say they're increasing the antibiotics; you'll continue them for a while once you're discharged. From home."

"You're sending him home with *pills*?" Deirdre looked up, straight at Monty.

"Absolutely not, Deirdre. No. Not pills. We'll put in a central line, and you'll hook the antibiotics up to him twice or three times a day, just like here."

Sheila leaned discreetly over to Deirdre, whispered in warning: "He's one of the good ones. There aren't many." Deirdre nodded back down to her book.

"What about the pain?"

"We've got people who deal with that. It'll be managed."

"So many people," Deirdre said. "Who's managing *them*? Who's overseeing all of this? Phelps doesn't seem to be."

"That," said Monty, "is a very good question." He seemed to ponder it, looked down at Patrick's file, began leafing through it, searching for something.

In the silence that followed, Deirdre continued writing; Sheila stepped out of the room; Patrick began worrying the base of the little tree with his right thumb. Jonathan stood stock still, then pronounced, as if it were the key: "So, Doctor, is he going to be alright?"

Patrick looked up. "Dad, I don't think …" He softened his gaze, looked down at his knees. "I don't think they *know*."

"We *never* know," Monty mumbled, still looking through the file.

An hour later, Patrick had finished dinner and was watching the news on television. Deirdre was sitting next to the bed, reading through her notebook.

Jonathan had gone back to his hotel for the night. Sheila was at the nurses' station, getting ready to end her shift, closing out her notes. Doctor Montgomery scuttled into the room, papers in both hands.

"Who is this ... Doctor Pettle? Works at the university? Came to visit Patrick a few times?"

Deirdre looked up. "I don't remember. Patrick?"

"He's a doctor at the clinic. I've seen him before, that time I had strep throat. Another time for a sprain. He came to visit? He must have heard I was sick."

"Do you like him?" Monty asked. "Do you get along with him?"

"Yeah, I think so. He's a nice guy. Older. He listens. I had a good conversation with him once. About Quakers."

"Quakers?" Deirdre asked.

"He's from an old Quaker family, back east. He works at the university. His wife's a doctor, too."

"I think I've met him," Monty said. "Can't remember where. Do you trust him?"

"Do I trust him? I don't know. With what?"

"You need a primary care doctor to take control of your case. Talk to doctors for you. Oversee. Make sure everything's in line. Follow up."

Deirdre sat up, alert, suddenly slightly relieved. "A primary care doctor."

"Yes. There's no one in charge right now. You're having to manage all of this yourself, and—no offense, Deirdre, really, you're wonderful, doing such a great job, but—you don't have the experience or the expertise to know how to talk to everyone. Just feeling your way through, trying to get a grasp of things. You need someone else, a doctor, someone who knows, to oversee everything. Manage it all."

"And this ..." she paused, looked down. "What's his name?"

"Doctor Pettle."

"Doctor Pettle could do that?"

"Well, I don't know. You'd need to ask him. But he's come to visit Patrick, which tells me he's paying attention. Got you on his brain."

"How do we find him?"

Monty rustled through the papers. "There's no number here. Call the clinic at the university. See if you can get him."

Deirdre wrote.

"And while you're at it, have him give me a call, will you?" He scribbled on a business card. "I'm going to leave you my private office number. *Don't* try to get me through the hospital switchboard. They'll just send you to an answering service. Have him call me here." He handed Deirdre the card, looked her in the eye. "*You* have been doing an *extraordinary* job, Deirdre. I mean it." He nodded at her, turned back to Patrick. "OK, champ. I'll be back tomorrow to check on you. Keep that hip dry, OK? And let it rest. Let it rest."

"I will. Thank you."

"You bet. Hang tight, I'll see you tomorrow."

"Good night."

It had started raining, a soft patter of tiny drops on the window, distorting the view beyond. Deirdre turned to watch it, thinking of whether or not she could go for a run. Patrick watched it, too, as much as he could.

"I don't know what to do, mom."

They continued watching the rain.

"I'm starting to feel—strange. I'm tired of people telling me how I should have died, like that somehow makes me strong and good."

"You *are* strong, Patrick."

"I don't feel strong. I feel tired."

"I know you do."

"How can I feel so tired when all I do is sleep and lie here? Useless."

"*Patrick.*"

"I mean it. How am I supposed to do this?"

"I'm here to help you."

He sighed. "I know."

Deirdre turned to look at him. She saw that something had changed: his face had relaxed in a troubling way; his eyes had lost focus, the muscles around them turned down like a frown. Like a lamp on a dimmer switch flickering at the lowest setting. Like a suit, off its hanger, crumpled on the floor. He reached for the wand that would deliver more pain meds into him, pressed its button. He closed his eyes, squeezed them shut, then released. He squeezed them again. A line of water spilled out from the right one, the most damaged one. It tipped round his cheek, then slid back to his neck, behind his ear. It seemed to dry instantaneously, as if in a desert, leaving only her knowledge that it had once been there.

"It did occur," she thought, "it did occur."

19

"Negative," Jonathan said. "Did you hear? It was negative."

"I heard," said Deirdre.

"Hallelujah. Oh, Deirdre. Some good news at last." His eyes were expansively hopeful.

Deirdre allowed for a small smile to cross her lips. "Yes, I guess so."

"Does he know?"

"Of course. They talked to him first. He had to sign something to allow them to tell us."

"He must be ecstatic."

"But he already knew it would be negative."

"Still. He must be beside himself. Some good news, Deirdre! I really think this is a turning point."

"I hope so," she said, not wanting to get caught up in his enthusiasm, but not wanting to dampen it, either. "I sure hope so."

The first time he went home, it was a bright but crisp day. Earlier that morning, he received news of the test results with a shrug, shook it off, and then began to arrange things on his lap: a few books, pairs of socks, some papers, the tree. He ordered them neatly, then rearranged them twice.

Sheila had given him one final burst of morphine, then removed the IV needle from his arm. The port from a central line, which threaded down to his heart from its heavily-patched entry point near his collar bone, dangled under his shirt. He was antsy, eager to go, but nervous, unsure what would await him outside. He did not know how long it had been since he had been brought to this place. It seemed like years.

"We're waiting on transport to take you downstairs," Sheila said, "and then you're a free man."

About a week had passed since Doctor Montgomery's surgery. In that time, he had been subjected to the widest possible range of imaging, all in the extended attempt to view and map the intricacies of bacterial itineraries, to seek them out and pinpoint their locations. The MRI—the most excruciating of these machines—had yielded little. Its dull, loud whizzes and pops translated inflammation into an image; but it could not see them. X-rays hinted that they might have entered some bone, but this hint was so subtle that the interpreters hadn't caught it. The grandest of all the techniques—a nuclear scan—gave a stronger sense of their presence. In the image (which Patrick was staring at now), their clusters looked like splotchy fields scattered around: pelvis, hip, leg, back. Compared to an earlier version, this one was plainer, quieter. The doctors decided this was good enough; it suggested to them that the war was being won. Only Deirdre had considered another rendering:

"But they're still there," she had said.

"Yes, but look at it next to this one. See how much smaller those blotches are? And they aren't in his organs anymore."

"What if they spread? Shouldn't he stay until they're all gone?"

"If only," one doctor had said. "If only we had enough beds and rooms and staff to keep everyone until they were totally done healing! We wish we could, Miss."

"Yes," said another. "And it'll be good for him to be home. Studies have shown that people heal faster in their own environment, where things are familiar."

"But they're still there," she said. "Even *I* can see them."

"Don't worry," the first doctor said. "We'll be in touch. And he'll have daily visits from home care. We'll keep working on it." Ironically—but with no sense of the irony—she said this as she slipped the image into a manila folder, slid it under a stack of similar folders, and folded her hands on the desk.

Deirdre scribbled in her book.

When the wheelchair arrived in Patrick's room, Sheila and Deirdre worked together to slide him over off the bed and down into the seat. He grimaced heavily; even with that last pool of morphine, he felt a stab in his back, an unhappy torque.

"OK?" Deirdre said once he was down.

"OK. Let's go."

Sheila leaned down to him, face-to-face. "I want you to stay away from here, OK? I never want to see you in that bed again. Stay away."

He smiled at her. "You won't miss me?"

"Others will take your place. Now go home. Finish getting better. You can come back *once*: when you're done with all this, and walk through that door just to bring me some flowers."

"OK," he said. "I will."

Sheila stood; and in an extremely uncharacteristic move, Deirdre wrapped her arms around her, squeezed hard, then held her shoulders as she smiled at her. She clenched her lips, then turned and walked out the door.

Down at the curb, the man pushing the wheelchair waited while Deirdre fetched the car. "Nice day," he said. "You think you can get up on your own? I got this back thing. Not supposed to lift."

"Mom can help me if I need it," Patrick said.

The car pulled up. Patrick grimaced again as he maneuvered himself, balancing first on the arms of the wheelchair and then on the rim of the door. He shifted carefully, choreographically. Deirdre kept a hand on the small of his back.

He was quiet for the first few minutes of the drive home.

"What are you thinking about?" Deirdre finally asked him, once she'd found the right throughway.

"I can't see the trees, mom. I can't see the trees." For the first time in so long he couldn't remember, Patrick began to weep, great heaving sobs from the bottom of him, from the bottom of everything, tearing up through his body like the spew from a long-dormant volcano. "Why can't I see the trees?"

And Deirdre wept with him. "I know, son. I know. It seems bad now. It won't seem this bad forever," she gasped between cries. "I promise, it won't." She reached over and grabbed his hand, squeezed it and held it that way. It was painful, a loving kind of pain that took the place, if only for a few minutes, of the unloving pain everywhere else.

This first time he went home was the worst. Once they had made it back to the flat, and moved Patrick and all his new paraphernalia into the front room, Deirdre sat down across from him and smiled. "Do you like the new chair? Your dad went and got it a few days ago. Thought it might be more comfortable than the other one."

"It is. It's huge. That was nice of him. Smart."

"Home care's going to be here in an hour. Someone named Diana. She's supposed to set us up with everything we need. She's some kind of supervisor. Someone else will be coming to visit every day. I can't pronounce her name. T-H-U-Y. How do you say that?"

"I think it's 'twee.' But we can ask her how she says it."

"How do you feel?"

"I think I'm in a lot of pain. Really stiff, but also like somebody's scooping something out of me."

"Let's see—they gave us some pills. I don't know if they're the same stuff that they had in the IV."

"This is ridiculous," Diana said later, once she'd arrived and was sitting between them. "These are basically aspirin. Here, Deirdre, take this prescription to the pharmacy while I'm sitting with Patrick. Tell them he was discharged today and it needs to be fast-tracked. They'll fill it while you wait, twenty minutes or so."

"Now?" Deirdre asked.

"Now."

Deirdre gathered her things, went quickly out the door.

"Are you a doctor?" Patrick asked.

"Nurse practitioner."

"You can write prescriptions?"

"Not for drugs like those. But I thought this might happen. It's common. So I dropped by the clinic and talked to Doctor Pettle between my last couple stops, had him write that just in case. He's gonna stop by later."

"Wow. Thanks."

"No problem. Gotta get the pain under control before we can do anything else. Wanna give me a number for your pain score? For my notes." She smiled as Patrick rolled his eyes. "I know, I know. But I've got to have something for the record."

"Right now, seven. Something like that."

"Got it. Where?"

He pointed to his left hip, then around to the lower part of his back.

"Now for me: what's it feel like?"

"Like someone's slowly chiseling out the inside of my leg."

Diana looked up, crossed her brow. "That does not sound fun."

"No."

They moved methodologically through the questions as Diana filled out the chart. Finally she put the papers away, leaned back, and smiled directly at him.

"OK. That's it. Now tell me. How are you doing?"

"I guess I'm fine. Everyone says I should be dead. Sometimes I wish I were."

"Don't blame you. But you're not. And that's a good thing, right?"

"Sure. Right."

"So let's keep it that way, OK?"

He snorted and smirked. "OK. Sure."

"You know what I mean by that?"

"Yes."

"I don't think you do. I've been doing this a long time, Patrick. Seen a lot of people in your situation. I know what to watch for."

"What's that."

"I don't need you to keep your spirits up all the time. You're going to feel pretty shitty about all of this sometimes, and that's fine. You're going to feel low. You're going to feel hopeless, like the cards are stacked so high against you, you can't see over them."

His eyes started to swell. "That sounds familiar."

"All of that is fine. It's normal. Feel bad sometimes. You have to. Why wouldn't you? This sucks. But you have to keep *wanting* to make it through. OK? Even when you feel like you won't, you need to keep *wanting*."

He nodded.

"OK? Deal?"

"Deal."

"When I got here, it looked like you'd forgotten that. Forgotten that you wanted to get through. I don't need to see that again. OK?"

"OK."

"And, Patrick, listen. This isn't a pep talk. I'm no good at those anyway. You're either going to make it, or you're not. Whether or not you *want* to make it, matters. It matters a great deal. I need you to remember that. You can't control most of this, but you can keep reminding yourself to want. It matters."

"OK."

"So tell me, do you want to make it through all this?

Patrick smiled—barely. "Yes. I do."

"Why?"

"What?"

"Why don't you want to die?"

He looked towards her harshly, like he'd been tricked, then softened his eyes, thought. A minute went by. "I want to travel again."

"Anywhere in particular?"

"Everywhere."

"What else?"

"I want to go out with my friends again. Have some drinks. Play pool. Flirt."

"Good. What else?"

"I want to have sex again."

"Who wouldn't. What else?"

"I want to watch the next Olympics."

"There you go. A good, specific goal—and not so far off. Excellent. What else?"

"I miss my cat. I want to adopt another cat."

"Yes. Go."

"I want to live here knowing that my mom is happily at home, *her* home, back east."

Diana smiled. "I bet she wants that, too. But let's keep that one to ourselves."

He laughed—really laughed, not long or hard, but still; he solidly laughed.

"So let's keep those things in mind, OK? Write them down even. It might sound silly, too simple. But it helps to have them at hand. For when you start feeling low—really low, you know what I mean. Might sound silly. But it works."

"I'll write them down."

"Good. Now let's talk about diet. I want you eating. A lot. Anything and everything you want. Do not hold back."

"What about the insulin?"

"You know how to use it, right?"

"Yeah, mostly."

"Stick to it. Dose according to what you eat, use the ratio the doctors worked out."

"Right."

"But eat. Eat everything you feel like eating." Diana paused. "You weren't diabetic before, huh?"

"No. They say the infection probably caused it somehow. Ate my pancreas. Think of that, at my age. Made me a ..."

"A *juvenile* diabetic, at *your* age. Good one." Diana had finished his joke for him. She smirked. "Not original, sorry." Patrick stared at her, caught mid-sentence. "And anyway, we don't call it juvenile diabetes anymore. It's Type 1." She smiled, a teacher's grin. "Does your mom cook?"

"Ha! Are you kidding?"

"She doesn't?"

"Mom hates to cook. She can make pasta with olive oil and she can reheat frozen vegetables. She can make a salad. She used to make these casseroles when I was a kid, but let's not talk about those."

"Got it. I'll talk to her about making sure you're eating."

"Good luck. She's not a big eater herself."

"What about exercise? You met with the physical therapist in the hospital?"

"Yes. He taught me what to do. Bend, flex; point, relax."

"Do those constantly. Not just to keep the muscles working, but also to keep the blood pumping. We don't want any clots."

"Right."

"Says here you were a gymnast? And a runner?"

"Yes. Gymnastics for twelve, thirteen years when I was younger. I've only been running the last few years. I did a marathon with mom last spring."

"That's good. Your body remembers. Just keep it moving, alright?"

"Alright."

Diana sifted through a few pages, turned them over and back again, then put the papers down and looked up. "OK, since you brought it up anyway, let's talk about sex."

Patrick looked at his hands.

"Anyone in the picture right now?"

He was tired. He could feel his leg, hollowing out.

"I'd just met someone. Right before. I don't know where that was going, but we were supposed to go out again."

"Have you talked to him since?"

"One of my friends called him. Let him know what was happening. He sent a really sweet card to the hospital, came by to visit once or twice. Said he was here to help."

"Lucky you. Sounds like a good one."

"I think so. He drives a tugboat. In the bay. Steers ships into port. We started calling him Tugboat Tim."

"Well! Hot."

Patrick smiled, snorted a short laugh. "I do alright."

"So here's the thing. Hips are messy, mixed up in an area with lots of other things going on. As you know. A kind of crossroads."

Patrick looked at her. "Yeah?"

"Yeah. You need to be careful down there. I'm not saying 'don't'; but should Tugboat Tim come knocking, just take it easy."

"I can't believe we're talking about this."

"Does it make you uncomfortable?"

"No, not like that. I just ..."

"You'd kind of forgotten about it? Forgotten your body is there for pleasure, too?"

"Something like that."

"A word of advice. Don't forget again. Helps with the wanting."

20

It was an unusually rainy December, cool and drenched. Aside from his view through the large plate-glass window in the main room of his flat, Patrick did not see much of the rain. He stayed mostly in the chair, wearing a path in the carpet between it and the bedroom or it and the loo. Deirdre relaxed into her caretaker role; she was doing some work, remotely, for her office back home, but otherwise sat with Patrick, tried to get him up and about, occasionally went for a run. She kept a calendar of visits, two or three a day, from friends in town. Some traveled in just to see him, worried from the updates they'd received on the massive mailing list set up by two of Patrick's closest friends, Robin and Jan.

Jan was the friend who'd found him that first day; through a bizarre coincidence, her mother had been in high school with Deirdre in Florida decades ago. (She remembered Deirdre as beautiful, popular, intimidating—all true.) So it was easy to get in touch, when Patrick was first taken to the ER. Thanks to Jan's assiduous calling, Deirdre had walked onto a flight from the east coast not three hours after Patrick was lifted onto a gurney and rolled away.

Robin, ten years older than Patrick, had become his scribe, his bellman, town crier. He sent regular missives to a growing list of people, keeping them up-to-date. He sat with Deirdre, joked with her, made her laugh. Elvish and wry, Robin was relentless in both optimism and glee. He brought bursts of energy to the wilted flat, like an electrical surge during a storm. He was here, now, helping Patrick as he continued to piece together the story.

"So you don't remember much of that day?"

"I remember waiting for Jan to get here for lunch. I remember what she looked like when she walked in, when she saw me, what state I was apparently in."

"Do you remember going to the clinic?"

"I remember parts of the ride. I was leaning against the window of the door, looking out. I remember seeing trees and the sky, in pieces."

"She took you to the clinic. They didn't know what to do, couldn't handle you. They called the ambulance."

"I don't really remember that."

"Do you remember the ER?"

"Bits and pieces. I remember waiting on a gurney in a hall. People looking down at me. I remember being rolled into a room, people rushing around, someone looking down and telling me to stop cracking jokes. I don't remember the jokes."

"You said, 'If you're going to go all *ER* on me, you could at least bring in Noah Wylie.' One of the nurses wrote it down." He chuckled at length.

"That sounds like me."

"Do you remember that first night in Critical Care?" As so often happened, Robin slid gracefully from laughter to sentimentality, began to well up.

"Just one thing. I remember feeling like I had to pee. It was the worst feeling. And no one would come to help me. That's it."

"You don't remember me?"

"You were there?"

"I got there late. Jan called, completely freaked out. I rushed over, but they'd already taken you into that glassed-in room, no outsiders allowed in. I watched you through the glass. I waved at you a couple times, thought you saw me before you were out."

"I might have. I don't know. I don't remember."

Robin wiped his eyes under his glasses, looked down. "Oh, honey, I thought we were losing you. Thought you were gone. They said you were going to die. I'd almost broken down when driving, had to pull over halfway across the bridge. I had Gary on the phone. You know how he is. Got all serious: 'Robin, *stop it*. This is what you have to do. Go to the hospital, be with him. He needs you there. Stop crying.' I told him I didn't know how I could handle it. He told me to shut up, start the car, and keep driving."

"You stopped in the middle of the bridge?"

Robin chuckled again. "Yes, honey, and it was *scary*. People were swerving all around me. Like in a windstorm, just because I'd stopped."

Patrick smiled at him. "You kind of *are* a windstorm."

Robin kept chuckling, continued: "What do you remember next?"

"Terrible things. They can't have been real."

"Like what?"

"People hunting me, or hunting something inside of me. Really hunting, with weapons. A room that was designed to change shape, to become a myriad of other rooms, constantly shifting. It was a modernist room once, all clean lines and beautiful chairs. And then a French boudoir, designed for sex, ornate and oily. And then a room by the sea, open and airy, linen drapes drifting with wind, teak chairs on a veranda."

"Sounds beautiful, interesting."

"It was horrible. Couldn't trust the room or anything in it."

"What else?"

"A deep blank. Not *nothing* exactly, just—absence, silence, darkness. I could tell there were things and people beyond it, but they were closed to me, unavailable. No, that's not quite right." He paused. "It's hard to describe."

"What else?"

"Oh, God, I forgot about the worst part. I think it was just before the first time I woke up, I'm not sure. I know I was out. Or at least I *hope* I was. I was at the top of a large, concrete coil—like the Guggenheim in New York, you know? Exactly like that, actually. Probably modeled on it."

"And what happened?"

"I was lying on a moveable bed. Not like a gurney; more a platform connected to a track, threaded into the walls of the coil. A large, complex system:

the track moved the platform, me on it, slowly down the path of the coil. There were large blades along the way, like meat slicers in a deli, only huge. Circular, spinning, arranged horizontally all the way down."

Robin uncrossed his legs, crossed them again with the other one on top.

"Each time I came to one, it slowly sliced away a thin layer of me. *Really* thin, like a micrometer thick. Someone, a man in a lab coat, explained to me that this is what happens when you die. Your body, every part of you, is slowly sliced away, disassembled in layers, then sent out to be reassembled with other pieces, from other people, somewhere else."

Robin gave a sharp intake of breath, like a gasp but less dramatic.

" 'This will be painful,' the man said. 'I'm sorry about that, but there's no other way.' The worst part was, the platform moved so slowly, so you could feel the slicers at work, feel the incisions. They took forever to shear away the pieces. Each layer like that. The man never explained *why* it was so slow, protracted."

"Oh, honey."

"I remember asking him, 'Will I remember? Will I remember who I am, or was? Will I remember *this*?' He just looked down at me, sad but clinical eyes, shook his head. So I started trying to remember everything I could. As the slicing was going on, I called up every single thing I could remember. Frantically, like packing a bag when you're late for a trip. I made myself remember: toys I had as a child, people I've known, the things I've done. Everything I could." He was briefly aware of the complexity of this moment: sitting here with his closest friend, trying to remember the remembering.

"Jesus, Patrick."

Patrick shrugged. He could still feel the feeling of that place, but had lost the emotional connection. He looked down, shrugged again.

Robin sighed, shook his head. He reached over and grabbed Patrick's hand. "Let's stop for now, OK?"

"Sure."

"Tugboat Tim's on his way over anyway."

"Do you think he knows we call him that?"

"Oh yes," Robin said. "I call him that to his face. Lots of other things I'd like to call him, too." He raised an eyebrow and smirked.

"Like what?"

"Use your imagination." He brushed off his lap, started to stand up. "So let's get you ready. Hair looks OK, could use a brush. Did you moisturize?"

"Bring me the lotion? It's by the sink."

"Wanna change your shirt?"

"No thanks."

"You sure? How about a blue one."

"Fine."

Robin went about the business of getting Patrick ready, chatting aimlessly about someone he had met on the train, a dog in the park, some shoes he wanted to buy. Patrick participated, not quite detached but not fully inside. "Could you bring me those pills? On the table. The biggest bottle."

"In pain?"

"Not too much. They say I've just got to stay on top of it. Take these on schedule, to keep it at bay."

"Your mom left a chart ..."

"It's in the notebook next to the pills, last page."

"And what do I do? Write it down?"

"Just check it off in the right box."

"Oh. Right, I see. Got it."

Patrick swallowed the pill, sat back in the chair. "Hey, you think you could help me get up for a few minutes? Before this kicks in. I want to walk around for a minute. Maybe go outside, get a breath of fresh air."

"You sure?"

"Yeah, I need to get up. I feel antsy."

"I'd feel antsy, too, baby, with Tugboat Tim on the way."

Robin reached around Patrick's back, the way Deirdre had shown him. He pulled a gentle pressure outward, away from the chair—not forcing Patrick up, but encouraging him in the right direction. Patrick pushed down on the arms, steadied his feet. As he started to rise, a sudden lightness hit him, not unpleasant, like the sandy shiftiness you feel when you first set foot on a ship. This lightness was followed, in quick succession, by a slight twist in his back, and then a sharp bolt up and down his left side. He gasped and slumped.

"Far enough! Far enough—*dammit*." He sat and leaned back. "Uh. Holy hell. I must have waited too long to take that pill."

"It's OK, honey, just relax." Robin placed his hand on Patrick's shoulder, kneeled down so he was eye-level. "It's OK. You're OK."

"*Jesus*."

"It's OK."

"I really wanted to get up."

"We'll do it later. Once the meds have kicked in, OK?"

"Yeah."

"What do you need?"

"Nothing. I'm fine. Just waited too long to take that damn pill."

"How long does it take to start working?"

"I can usually feel it relaxing me in twenty, thirty minutes."

"Just in time for Tim. Good. You OK?"

"I'm OK. Hey, why don't you put on some music. Something chipper. No guitars."

Robin started playing disco, his usual call. Patrick let its buoyancy drift over and around him, softening him. He wondered how long it would be before this stopped feeling normal again. As Robin danced around the kitchen, putting things away, Patrick reached over to his right side, felt for the paper, brought it up: the list. Travel, he would think about travel. No, playing pool—Robin could help with that.

"Hey, remember that night I met Ryder?" he called to the kitchen.

"At the Pils? You bet I do. You were a shark that night. Like there were hole-magnets in the balls."

"Let's go play again soon. I miss it."

"You got it, baby," Robin called, swaying in the other room, "you got it."

21

He had stopped dreaming.

Nights were hard, bitter, cold, and got progressively worse. Deirdre would help him get settled, tuck him in like a child; and then he would lie for at least an hour, listening passively to an audiobook or thinking aloud. By 1 a.m., he and his sheets would be drenched, the tide of night sweats so high, so insistent, that finally Deirdre bought and installed an absorbent sheet, made for bed-wetting five-year-olds. The indignity of it soured him on sleep, so that he started dreading the arrival of bedtime with viscous intensity, clinging to the minutes in late afternoon and evening with a desperate anxiety, willing them to expand so as to hold off the night. Eventually he would succumb, drifting off into a soft kind of stoic worry: maybe it would be different tonight—maybe; but no, of course it won't. It never is. Then in bed, he would wait for the sweating to start again, resigned to the inevitable wakings, the calls to Deirdre, her lifting him up to dry his back and legs.

This was why he had stopped dreaming. It was as if the worry filled what sleep he got so fully that there was room for nothing else, not even rest. In the mornings, already awake as light slowly stirred the room, he would roll partway onto his side, wait for the sound of Deirdre pattering into the bathroom before she peeked in on him.

"You awake?" she'd always say. The only beauty of mornings, for him, was that night would be then so far off.

"His sed rate's still high. Way too high," Diana said, looking closely at a print-out of his most recent lab results. "It had started coming down, but it's shot up again."

On this particular morning, Diana had made a special trip to see Patrick; Doctor Pettle had come, too, and sat now on a chair dragged into the room from the kitchen table. "I see that. His CRP is high, too."

"What's the CRP again?" Deirdre asked, writing.

"C-Reactive Protein. Another test for infection," Doctor Pettle said. "Both of these results are very high, which suggests an active infection. A normal sed rate, for example, should be below 15. Patrick's is over 100."

Patrick sat in his chair. He was scratching a spot on his left arm, near the elbow, where something had chaffed. "What does the sed rate measure again?"

"It means 'sedimentation rate.' After we draw your blood, we measure how long it takes for the red blood cells to fall, to drift down and rest at the bottom of the sample. When there's an active infection at work, blood cells start to stick together, so they fall faster."

"And mine are falling very fast."

Doctor Pettle smiled gently, "Yes, that's exactly right."

"So what do we do?"

"Well, there are few things we know. Your sed rate went down initially, once you got home. It had been this high, and then it went to 80, then 60, then 40. That tells us that something was working—probably a combination of the high dose of antibiotics, everything they'd done in the hospital, and, well, your robustness. You should feel good about that."

"Can I hold off on feeling good about that until this is all done?"

"Of course, of course. We also now know that your sed rate shot back up very quickly, in a matter of days. Something changed, the bacteria took stronger hold, and have very quickly begun to spread again. Most likely," he cautioned prudently, "most likely. We aren't sure. Of course it's possible that this is just an aberration, a trick result."

"What do *you* think?"

Doctor Pettle removed his glasses, rubbed the bridge of his nose, and then threaded them back on, their stems wrapping over and around his ears. "I don't want to take any chances. I wish they had not discharged you before the sed rate was in normal range. I think we need to go back to the hospital."

Diana sighed deeply and closed her eyes. When she opened them again, she said, "I agree. I'm sorry, Patrick, but I just don't think they've got to the root of this thing."

Deirdre began flipping through her book. "What was his sed rate when they discharged him?" They all began leafing through their notes, except Patrick, who was staring at the window. "Wait, here it is. It was 82? Can that be right?"

Doctor Pettle read from his file. "82. Yes, I have that, too. That's really high."

"And they discharged him anyway?"

Doctor Pettle sighed. "I'm afraid so. I would have made a different decision, I think. But they likely had good reason to believe he was truly on the mend. It's not as uncommon as I would hope."

"You know what," Patrick suddenly said, "you know what? I don't want to dwell on this, whether or not they should have sent me home. They *did*, end of story. And I'm not getting better. So let's just go back."

"Well," Doctor Pettle said quickly, "it's not quite that simple. We have to find a bed. You can't just walk back into the hospital and get a room. You have to make arrangements."

"Arrangements?" Deirdre asked, "Like a hotel? That's ridiculous."

"I know. It is." Doctor Pettle paused, looked down at his file, thought carefully. "Let me suggest this. I suspect, based on these images, that the infection may have moved into his bone. It's faint; but right here near the thigh, there's something going on in there. Let me call someone in orthopedics, get him in for a visit. If someone there can confirm a bone infection, they'll get him a room pronto. They'll need to act quickly."

"How soon can we get in to see someone?" Deirdre asked.

"Let me go call now. I'll try for today, OK?" He rifled through his bag for the phone, then walked out the front door to the balcony there, where the others could eventually hear his soft voice in conversation with others.

Robert Pettle was a small, delicate man, with pointed features and an immensely unpretentious manner. He reminded Patrick of a character from a childhood book: The Littles—he even looked like he might have a small tail. And he was unlike any of the other doctors Patrick had met: soft-spoken, genuinely kind, empathic—but in a way that assumed neither too much nor too little. He was whip-smart, a trait he had demonstrated in navigating between the many offices he called on Patrick's behalf; but his manner was so calm, so conversational, so affectionately engaged, that it was generally only in retrospect that you realized how very smart he was.

They could hear him, now, speaking more insistently than they'd ever heard him be before. "No, *today*," he said. "This afternoon. It is *urgent*. ... Yes, urgent.... No, I'm sorry, I'm afraid that won't work.... I see.... Yes, I see. Listen, would you please put me through to Doctor Shin's office phone? As I said, we've worked together on a complex case before, and perhaps he'll be able to find some room.... Yes, of course. I understand. You can't just create time. But, please, this really is terribly urgent.... Thank you so much. I appreciate it. You've been very helpful. Thank you."

Eventually, after speaking with the doctor himself, he returned to the room with a hopeful—but not too hopeful—look on his face. "Some good news. We're going to see someone today, at 3. Doctor Michael Shin. He's an orthopedic surgeon, connected to the hospital. He's very good."

(Did anyone, Patrick thought, ever refer to a doctor as anything other than "very good"? But he let this pass.)

"Has he seen Patrick before?" Deirdre asked.

"No, but he knew of his case. You were big news, Patrick. You're famous there. Not that that's a good thing, I know. But in this case, it has helped."

In the thought that he might be immediately admitted back into hospital, Deirdre packed a small bag for Patrick before the appointment. Plenty of socks, a change of clothes, toiletries, a few books. She packed some photographs of friends, some cards he had been sent. She'd make a nice little display, she thought, opposite his bed. She packed herself a bag, too, for spending the night. She didn't need much.

Doctor Shin confirmed what Pettle had feared, expanded on its severity. It was after 5 p.m. "See, here?" He said, pointing to a spot on the X-ray from Patrick's file. "The bone is mottled, like lace. Just around the edges. That's the infection."

"This is the last X-ray," Deirdre asked, "from just before he was discharged?"

"Looks like it, yes. It's a very minor detail. Not unusual that they wouldn't have caught it. And all signs pointed to things being under control."

"But they weren't."

"Apparently not, or perhaps they just started up again. Hard to say."

"What about now?"

"Yes. So. I'll need to do another X-ray."

"Can we do it today?" It was Monday.

"I'm afraid not, no. We'll do it Wednesday."

"Doctor Shin, please, can't we just do it now?"

"No. I'm heading out now, and am out of the office tomorrow. I've already booked him for an appointment on Wednesday afternoon. It's fine, really. A couple nights won't hurt him." He turned to Patrick. "Go home tonight, sleep in your own bed, let's see what the X-ray shows us on Wednesday, OK?" Patrick did not respond. He was thinking about Berlin, wondering if the old tenement building housing artists—every room a makeshift studio—still stood. Wondering if he could see it again, next time he was there.

Deirdre sighed, looked at the floor. "What happens once we've done the X-ray?"

Doctor Shin leaned back on the ledge near the sink, crossed one arm across his waist, balanced the other on top of it and stroked his chin. "Well, if I can still see signs of infection, and especially if it's progressed, I'll need to operate. So let's say this: we'll do the X-ray on Wednesday afternoon, I'll take a quick look at it while you wait, and we'll plan to have you checked in to a room, do the surgery the following morning. That's Thursday."

Despite her impatient frustration, Deirdre was briefly calmed by having a schedule, something to expect. "OK," she said, "OK." She rocked slightly in the plastic chair, back-and-forth, back-and-forth, with something more than nervous energy and something less than general compulsion. She rocked as Doctor Shin went over details with Doctor Pettle, who had sat in silent witness for the latter part of the appointment. She rocked because it kept her from sinking; she rocked because it kept her from screaming. She rocked because if she hadn't, she might have torn the very plaster from these walls, spreading its crumbling dust across the tiles, out into the hall, and over on top of everything she could find.

22

"Suzanne, beware of the devil ..." Patrick was singing suddenly, almost in full voice. He wasn't sure where it had come from. "Don't let him spoil your heart." Deirdre had gone for a run, would be gone for an hour or more. Patrick was in the flat alone, lying down for once on the couch, his legs stretched out below him, crossed, rocking back-and-forth. "Suzanne, beware of the devil, don't let him pull us apart." He stopped, realizing that those were the only lyrics of the song he knew. He sang them again, and once again.

The sun was out. Filtered through the leaves outside the window, it spotted Patrick's face and body, breaking them up. He rocked his head back-and-forth, alternating the direction he rocked his legs, and watched the sun twinkle in and out, in and out. It had a strange effect: because his visual field was spotted, too, refusing any sense of a full image, the flickering sun and the fractal shadows cast by the leaves made his vision seem whole, obstructed externally rather than internally. It had surprised him when he first noticed it, and he enjoyed playing with it, giving it legs, as they say. It seemed to trick his brain somehow, and this lifted his mood. "Suzanne, beware of the devil," he sang again, "don't let him spoil your heart. Suzanne, beware of the devil—"

He was interrupted by a considerate knocking on the door, not too loud, not too soft. He lifted his head, yelled "Come in!" then began to shift himself around, bringing his feet to the floor. "Come on in!"

The door pulled away, replaced by a familiar voice: "How's the little prince today?" It was Tugboat Tim, dropping by on his way home from work. Patrick watched as Tim's head came into view: the black, curly hair sculpted in place; the strong, rugged line where jaw met neck; the dark, sad eyes that would suddenly transform whenever Tim smiled.

"Fine, fine! Hi! Come on in! I didn't know you were coming over today. Done with work?"

"Yeah, slow day. Hey, look at you!" Tim reached down, grasped Patrick's head between his hands. They were rough, mealy: hands that had pulled a lot of rope. "You're looking extra good today."

"Liar."

"Am not! You're glowing a little. Feeling good?"

"Feeling OK. Nervous about tomorrow."

"Yeah. I bet." He put his arms around Patrick, squeezed then released. "What time is it happening?"

"We're supposed to go in at 4. Who knows when they'll get to me."

"OK. I'm gonna try to get off early, head over as quick as I can. I'll come straight through, won't need to stop at home."

"You don't have to do that."

"I want to. And somebody needs to be there to stop your mom from ripping that guy's head off."

"Oh man. She's *really* mad at him. Doesn't want me to know, but I heard her on the phone last night. I haven't heard her talk about someone that way since before she left dad."

"She told me. I called this morning, earlier, when you were napping. She sounded *dangerous*."

"Don't mess with Deirdre. She'll take you out."

"Yes she will." Tim pulled at the arms of his coat, lengthening them out. "So you're sitting over here today. Not too much pain, huh?"

"Nope, not too much. I think remembering to take the meds on time helps."

"Good, good. You hungry?"

"I could eat."

"So I had this idea—already mentioned it to Deirdre, so she won't worry if you're not here when she gets back. Why don't I drive you out to that burger place you like? You won't have to get out of the truck. I can get the food and bring it out, we can have a little picnic in the parking lot."

Patrick smiled a broad smile.

"Is that a yes?"

"That, my friend, is a yes."

"When did you take the last pill?"

"Couple hours ago. Why?"

"Maybe you should take another, just to be safe. Don't want you to lose this momentum."

"Good idea."

It took some maneuvering, and a bit of heavy lifting, to get Patrick into the truck. His leg still wasn't fully able to bear his weight, and the cab of the truck was high. Tim wedged himself between Patrick and the runner board, cranked him up like a jack.

"That was fun," Patrick sneered once they were on their way, his face twinkling with sweat.

"Focus on the burger. Focus on the fries. Twenty minutes and they'll be in your hands."

"Twenty-*three* minutes, and they'll be in my stomach." He wondered if he hadn't made a mistake. The truck's seats were not cushioned, and Tim's driving wasn't smooth. Patrick held his tongue, not wanting to spoil Tim's gesture, so thoughtful, so selfless.

"So, how you holding up?" Tim asked as they shot up the ramp to the freeway. "Woah, watch it buddy!" He was not generous with merging. The truck lurched to the right, then back to the left, as a small two-door swerved at an angle to pass them.

Patrick held on to the passenger door, knuckles blanched. "Oh—yeah, I'm holding up. Well, up and down. Today's been pretty good, calm before the storm."

"Calm before the storm. Maybe there won't *be* a storm."

"Maybe."

"You never know."

Patrick looked out the side window, watching for trees. They weren't quite out of the city yet. They drove in silence for a few moments. Tim was driving with his left hand, right arm draped back over the long bench-seat, hand on Patrick's shoulder.

"What does a tugboat actually do?" Patrick asked.

"Well, let's see. Mostly pulls other things around—ships, barges, platforms. Keeps things moving safely in tight spaces. Helps move things that have broken down."

"What did you move around today?"

"Not much tugging today, actually. They're planning an exercise for next week, big project, so we mostly worked with them on that."

"Who's they?"

"Bay officials, coast guard, environmental folks."

"Are you allowed to talk about it?"

"Oh yeah. They're worried about what would happen if a loaded container ship or an oil rig went dark in or near the bay. Lost power. Lots of currents out there, so lots of things could happen: it could just drift out into the ocean, which actually wouldn't be the worst to deal with. It could run into a pylon, one of the bridges. Could hit another ship, or could crash into the land. Those are some big problems right there."

"And they're working with environmentalists?"

"Oh yeah. Nothing happens in San Francisco without them."

"What are they worried about? Oil and gas leaks?"

"Yep, but that's not all. They're worried about the Headlands. In Marin."

"Everybody's always so worried about Marin. What about Oakland?"

Tim chuckled. "Nobody ever says too much about Oakland. All that coastline along the Headlands, those are delicate—what do you call them? Ecosystems. Delicate ecosystems."

"Delicate ecosystems," Patrick said wryly.

"Yep. They're worried about a ship crashing into them, disturbing things."

"I guess that's noble. I'd be more worried about Oakland. We're a delicate ecosystem over here, too, you know."

"Spoken like an Oaklander."

"Damn straight. So what's the exercise? What are they going to try?"

"They're going to get a fully loaded container ship, six or seven levels high, put it in the middle of the bay, and turn it off."

"Turn it off? Just like that?"

"Yep. Shut 'er down."

"Then what?"

"Two tugs, one in front pulling, the other in back pushing, will move the ship in towards the shipyards. Then they'll stop it, hold it there. And then the trickiest part: turn the ship around and move it back."

"*Turn it around?*" Patrick asked, gaping at Tim.

"Yep."

"Two little tugboats?"

"Yep."

"Can you *do* that?"

"Oh yeah. We'll be able to do it. But it's tricky."

"Wow. And you'll be in one of the tugboats?"

"Oh yeah. I'm captain of the lead."

"Seriously?"

Tim smiled, turned to Patrick. "You know, I'm pretty good at what I do."

"Oh, I know, I mean, I figured. Sorry, I didn't mean—"

Tim chuckled, "Don't worry. It's OK."

"I'm just—wow. It sounds so intense, so ... delicate. As a maneuver."

"It is."

"I'm really impressed."

"Don't be impressed yet. I'll let you know how it goes next week."

Patrick thought about this, imagined the scene, seeing Tim in a tiny white boat yanking a massive barge with a rope. It was utterly unfathomable except in the most pedestrian sense: like a cartoon, little boats with smiling faces, tooting horns. He could not even begin to think through how it all must work, drew a complete blank—nothing.

"You really are a tugboat captain."

"I really am."

Rested and full, Patrick sat on his chair, back at the flat, while Deirdre and Tim looked through some papers that had just arrived in the post. "I don't understand," Deirdre said. "What does it mean?"

"I think we need to call them." Tim's brow was deeply furrowed as he tried to parse some complicated prose printed in miniature font. "How are you supposed to *read* this? I've got 20/20 and I can barely make it out."

"Where's your insurance card? I can't find it."

"I think you put it back in my wallet, mom. Over on the bookshelf," Patrick replied, trying not to get too involved.

She fetched the wallet, found the card and pulled it. "This is regular insurance, right? Like mine?"

"I don't know, mom. It came with grad school. They gave it to me when I started. I haven't thought much about it."

"Here, it says right here: '$500,000 lifetime maximum.' Right here on the back. Is that normal?"

"I have no idea."

"Is that a lot?"

"I don't think so," Tim said, "I don't think it is."

"And the letter says he's almost hit half of his lifetime maximum?"

"That's what it says."

"How is that possible?"

"I think we need to call them, Deirdre. You still have copies of all the bills? I think we need to look at those and then call them."

"Can we look at this stuff later?" Patrick asked. "I know it's important. I just don't want to get all riled up tonight. Can we put it away for now?"

"Of course we can, son. Good, let's put it away. Tim, can you hand me that folder? The blue one."

Still trying to make out the text on the letter, Tim glanced up and seemed to give Deirdre a meaning-filled look, seemed to talk to her through the eyes. He held her gaze for a few seconds; she nodded, almost imperceptibly, then reached out her hand. Tim turned the pages over, shook them together into place, and handed them and the folder to her. She tidied them all and slid them into her bag on the floor, patted it twice, then looked up with a tight smile. "What now?" she said. "Movie?"

Patrick's dreams were back. He credited Tim, for obvious reasons: in this one, Patrick wore yellow rain bibs, just the bottoms, as he waded through a shallow pool. The water was clear, like clean cellophane draped a foot above neat patterns of rocks and stones, rainbows of sand, tiny glycerin fish darting around in short straight lines. He leaned down to watch them and followed the patterns they took: each one seeming to trace out a square, slightly off-kilter, with its little jumps forward. His vision had been clear in previous dreams, as if nothing had happened to his eyes. But in this one, the now-familiar pocks of dark absence had started to appear. He stood and turned to look behind him, over his right shoulder, and saw the opening to a cave. And then, in a flash, his view toggled, as if he were in the cave—or, no, as if he *were* the cave—watching himself stand in the pool. He thought, "How strong he looks, that man there. How lithe. How unlike others who have come before. That man there shouldn't have seen me. He shouldn't have noticed me at all."

23

The dream had not been unpleasant; but Patrick awoke with a deepened sense of complexity, feeling that the shape of things to come was more elaborate, more ornate, than he was comfortable realizing. It was not a foreboding feeling exactly, more like a studied appreciation of the baroque.

Deirdre was already up and about, shifting things around in the other room. It sounded like she was moving heavy things, like furniture. "Mom?" he called.

He heard her pause, then walk to his room. "Hey! Ready to get up? I'm just making a few changes in here."

"What are you doing?"

"Just moving some things around. Changing things up. It's been feeling stale. We'll see if you like it. If not, I'll put it all back."

"I'm sure it's good. I'm ready to get up."

Because he could not shower, Patrick had become accustomed to a morning convention that still felt surreal: he would stand, balancing himself by holding onto the sink, while Deirdre helped him bathe with a steaming washcloth. He had stopped feeling humiliated, but he still felt out of place in it, and each time tried to blank it out from his memory as soon as it was done. She was crouched down behind him now, washing his legs.

"What's this scar? Right here, near your shin. On the left."

Patrick looked down, tried to find what she was talking about. He reached and felt with his right hand until he tracked down the spot. It had been a small, oval wound, about a half-inch at its widest diameter. "Oh—that. Right. I think that was a burn. I bumped into something, a really strong lamp. It burned me."

She inspected it closely. "I didn't notice it before."

"Wasn't a big deal. Took a while to heal."

"Did it hurt?"

"Yeah, actually, it did. I was supposed to run the Wharf-to-Wharf about a week after it happened. But I couldn't because it was still swollen. Had to keep my leg elevated instead."

"I don't remember you telling me about that," she said, still looking closely. "What's the Wharf-to-Wharf?"

"Sort of like Bay-to-Breakers, but in Santa Cruz. Fewer hills."

"Oh. Never heard of it," she said, moving on. "I'll step out while you do the rest." She went, closing the door behind her.

He washed himself, front then under and back, trying not to let the work of it settle too far into him. He took his time, careful to get to everything. When he had finished with the first pass, he turned and rinsed the cloth, watching the hoary water circle the drain and go in. He turned the hot water up, drenched the cloth, and cleaned again.

When he was done, Deirdre helped him get to his chair. She had moved it closer to the window, which he appreciated, circling the other pieces around, on one side towards the kitchen, on the other towards the front door. It threw him, for a moment, and he paused to map it all, willing himself to remember where things were. "Looks good," he said.

"I think it takes better advantage of the light," Deirdre said, "coming in from the window. Coffee? Thuy called. She's on her way."

"Yes, thanks. When will she be here?"

Thuy Nguyen was the regular home care nurse, a daily visitor for the weeks Patrick had been home. She was tall—almost as tall as Patrick—and excruciatingly thin. Her voice was both light and sharp, occupying the highest registers Patrick had ever heard in everyday speech. And she was enormously bubbly, wickedly clever, exceedingly nice. He liked that she came every day, and would sit listening to her talk about what she called her *pickles*: boy trouble, friend trouble, mother trouble.

"I've got a pickle again," she said after she'd arrived and set up. She threaded his arm through a black cuff and began pumping the rubber balloon. "With Rob. I just don't get it." She paused, listening.

"What'd he do?" Patrick asked.

Thuy seemed to ignore him for about half a minute as she watched the dial, air gradually releasing from the cuff. "One-seventeen over seventy—great!" She undid the Velcro, pulled the cuff away. "He's going on a trip for work, to Orlando. They're sending him there to meet with some people about insurance or something, I don't really know. They're sending him with this woman he works with—Patrick, he used to *date* her. For like eight months. And he wanted to know if I would mind if they shared a hotel room. '*Double beds*,' he kept saying, 'a room with *double beds*.' "

"Why would they need to share a room?" Patrick asked.

"He works for a start-up. They're trying to save money. He kept telling me about these beds, like that was the most important detail. 'Rob,' I said. 'Listen.' " She drifted away for a moment as she reached for a thermometer and stuck it in Patrick's mouth. "Under your tongue." She jotted something down quickly in her notes. " 'Rob,' I said, 'stop talking about the beds. I'm not comfortable with you sharing a room.' Nice and clear, you know? Just like I'm supposed to. 'I'm not comfortable' with whatever rather than 'No, you can't.' " Thuy had been seeing the same therapist for weekly sessions over the past few years, a fact of which she reminded Patrick every time she visited. She was working on communicating her needs without being overbearing, as she put it.

"Sounds good to me," Patrick mumbled as best he could with the thermometer sticking out.

"I mean, we're getting *married* in four months. We're having a *wedding*. And he wants to share a hotel room in Florida with some ex? Give me a *break*." She plucked the thermometer out, looked at it, wrote down what it said. "Everything looks good here. I just need to take some blood. Diana thinks we should have a record of where things are before you're back in the hospital."

"OK."

"Just—let me see—two vials, I think." She scanned her notes. "Yeah, two. The basics."

"OK."

"God, you have such good veins. Mine are so tiny. They can never find them."

"Yeah, I've heard that before."

"I mean look at this one! Like it's just begging to have me stick something into it!"

He laughed, said, "When we were training to do phlebotomy, when I volunteered at the free clinic, everybody always wanted to practice on me their first time. Before they tried harder veins. I got stuck so many times, it was crazy. Had a permanent bruise for a while."

"I forgot you did that. Up in Berkeley?" She wrapped a tourniquet around his left arm, tightened it.

"Yeah."

She wiped the inside corner of his elbow; she bent to insert a butterfly needle, taped it down, popped a vial on the other end of its tube. Quick and easy, not giving it a second thought. A thin red line made its way from arm to glass, dripping then spurting a steady flow. She waited a moment until it filled, then pulled it off, tipped it back-and-forth to mix it, and replaced it with a second vial. After a few seconds, she pulled the tourniquet loose and told him to relax his arm. She had a particular way of doing this, tracing her nails down his palms and along his fingers as she spoke. He liked the feeling. It worked to resolve the tension from the draw, to let it go.

"So you're going back today. Good luck, Patrick. Really, I'll be thinking about you. I'll send you good vibes, OK? Get out soon so I can visit you again. I'm taking a leave starting late March."

"I'll do my best. Maybe it won't be more than a few days. Maybe it won't even be that long."

"Don't think in numbers. Don't think in length. Just get better, OK?"

She leaned over and gave him a quick kiss on the cheek before she left, looked at him full-on, grinned and said, "Get better for the boys. I'm sure they miss you out there."

"Good luck with Orlando."

"Rob's the one needs the luck." She shot him a look before turning and going out the door, and he could hear her stomping heavily as she made her way along the balcony and down the open stairs.

24

"I'm mad at you," Sheila said, walking into the room. "I told you I didn't want to see you in here again."

"Hey, Sheila! Are you my nurse?" Patrick said, happy to see her.

"Yep. I'm still upstairs, but they asked me to work down here while you're in. Wanted to give you some familiarity, make it a bit more comfortable. OK with you?"

"Completely OK. Great!" he said.

"Plus, Aamir's on this ward now. He's going to stop in to say hi in a bit."

"Really? I brought his tree."

"I see that. How you feeling?"

"Nervous. But kind of excited too, like something good might happen."

"Keep thinking that way. That's what we want to see. How's your pain?"

"Not bad: three or four. I took a pill before I left home."

"When? An hour ago?"

"More than that. They had us waiting downstairs for a while. It's probably been three hours."

"Right. Let's get you hooked up quick, then. You remember this?" She held up the wand. "Remember how it works?"

"Yep. My old friend. I remember him well."

"Why's it gotta be a he?" Sheila asked.

Patrick laughed. "My mom asked me that once. 'Why's it gotta be a he?' I answered honestly. She's never asked again."

Sheila smiled. "Where *is* Deirdre, by the way?"

"Went to get some food. We were waiting a long time."

"Your dad still here?"

"No. He went home after I was discharged last time. Said he'd come out if I need him to. I told him to wait, see what happens."

"Good. He tenses your mom right up."

"Oh, you don't have to tell me. Welcome to the first thirteen years of my life."

"Ooh. Seriously. Some people just should *not* be in the same room."

"You got that right." He bristled at the thought of all the rooms they *had* been in together over the years, felt the start of a defensive shield rising.

She looked at his file. "They did the X-ray?"

"Yeah, a little while ago. Said they'd send the images straight to Doctor Shin, right away. He's probably got them by now. I don't know how long it takes."

She flipped through the pages, then hooked the file back to its spot on the baseboard of the bed.

"OK. They've got you on a lower dose of pain meds than you were on before. If it's not enough, let me know. Early. Don't wait for the pain to take over."

"I won't. I wish I didn't need them at all."

She looked at him. "What do you mean?"

"I don't know. I feel like a junkie. I mean, I know I need them. I've felt what it's like to be in real pain, to try to get through it without them. I know I need them. But I wish I didn't. Probably good to have a lower dose, start to wean me off them."

Sheila pulled up a chair, sat down and leaned over to him. "Listen to me very carefully. I don't like hearing you use the word junkie." She took his hand. "You hear me? Do not use that word."

"OK, OK, I know I'm not a junkie, it's just—"

"No, listen. Someone explained this to me once in a way that makes sense. Imagine a swimming pool in the ground, made out of cement, surrounded by a tile patio. Got it?"

"Yes."

"The swimming pool is *you*. Now imagine rain, a heavy rainstorm over the pool. Got it?"

He nodded, thinking how nice it would be to swim.

"The rainstorm is the meds. People who are not in pain, their swimming pool is already full of water, filled right up to the top. Add the rain, and the pool spills over and floods everything, makes the patio slippery, makes everything unusable, dangerous."

"OK …"

"People who aren't in pain, if they take these meds, become dangerous. Nothing works right. Unusable. But people in pain: their pools are low, maybe getting empty. Not enough water. Dangerous. Add the rain, that level comes up. Makes the pool function again as it should, safe for swimming. Pool needs the rain. People in pain need the meds. Understand?"

"Yeah. I do."

"Your pool is empty. You need the rain."

For some reason, this made him suddenly tender. He was moved by her metaphor. "I need the rain."

"So no more talk about junkies."

"No more talk about junkies."

"Promise?"

"I promise."

"Good." She squeezed his hand, got up and moved the chair back against the wall. "Be back in a few minutes."

When Deirdre returned, she found places for the bags she had brought and began tidying up the room. Patrick was watching her work. "Hey mom," he said. "Do you want to sleep back at the apartment tonight? Would it be good for you to have some space to yourself? Nothing big is happening overnight. I'd be fine here alone."

"Thanks, Patrick, but I'd rather stay."

"OK. I like having you here. But it's OK with me if you need a break."

"I'll be fine. I'll pull one of those recliners in here again. They're actually pretty comfortable."

Doctor Shin walked into the room, carrying a clipboard stacked with papers. "Mister Anderson. You made it."

"Hi, Doctor Shin."

"Looks like Sheila's got you all set up. Need anything?"

"How are the X-rays?"

"I haven't seen them yet. They're probably back in my office. It's been a long day."

"When do you think you'll be able to let us know?" Deirdre asked. "We're curious about what's next."

"Of course you are, of course you are. I'm headed back soon, need to make just a stop or two more. Really busy day, actually. Haven't had a minute to catch my breath. I'll get to them as quickly as I can, come back and talk with you then."

"OK. Don't let us hold you up. We're fine here for now." She began setting up food on the tray near Patrick's bed, laying out the plastic flatware and napkins, moving things from boxes to a plate.

"What's for dinner?" Doctor Shin asked with a smile.

"Apparently it was meatloaf from the kitchen. I brought Patrick some lasagne."

"Sounds good! You must be quite the chef."

"I bought it, take-out," she said matter-of-factly.

"Right. Well, enjoy it, Patrick. I'll see you in a little while."

Patrick had begun to feel some anxious but happy anticipation. He wasn't sure why; but he had begun to develop a thought that this might be the night they would pinpoint the problem and map out a plan for treatment, one that wouldn't take too long. He began to feel buoyant, optimistic, strong. "Mom, can you hand me some paper and a pen?"

Deirdre was shocked. She looked at him. "Sure I can, hang on." She rustled through her bag, brought them out and lay them on his table. "What do you want to write?"

Aside from scribbling his signature across a few forms, he hadn't written since before this had all begun. It wasn't going to be easy to start again. He would have to learn to see the page again, to follow his writing, through or around the splotches his new vision had. "I've just been thinking about a few things. I want to write them down."

He wrote for several minutes without ceasing, achingly slow but steady: "So broken, so many parts of me. Finally feels there's a plan to put me back together again. First time in ages I've felt like I might have an *after* to this, an after to live in and fill out" was the opening bit.

When he had finished, he handed the paper and pen back to Deirdre. "I want to keep writing," he said, "but please promise me you won't read it. I want to work through some things, put some of this stuff running through my head down on paper. Get it out of me. I need to know it's private, OK?"

"I promise you," she said. "I will not read it."

It was early evening; the light coming through the window was all street lamps and moon, the winter sun having finished its work a while ago. There was a soft knock from outside the room. "Patrick? Deirdre? It's Aamir. Mind if I come in?"

Patrick sat up. His hand unconsciously went to his head, tousling his hair just so. "Aamir! Yes, please, come in!"

He entered humbly, hugging a file full of papers close to his chest. Deirdre was grinning wildly again. "Hi, Aamir. Looks like you couldn't get rid of us."

"Hi, Deirdre, Patrick. I can't believe you're back. I'm so sorry this is still happening." He actually looked concerned; he actually looked sorry. "When Sheila told me you were coming back, well." He walked to the bed, lay the file at its foot, then shifted and put a hand on Patrick's shoulder.

"Oh, it's OK. I basically insisted. They didn't finish, last time. I just want them to finish, to get it all. I'm feeling better, really. It's just not done yet."

"How are your spirits?"

"Better than the last time I saw you. I think this is it, you know? I feel like things are going to get better soon."

Aamir squeezed his shoulder, smiled. "You look fantastic. Like you've gotten some of yourself back."

"I feel like I have."

"Pain?"

"Yeah, that part hasn't been great. But it's under control."

"Got the button?"

"Right here. Actually ... thanks for the reminder. I haven't pushed it in a while."

"Stay on top of it, Patrick." He looked down sternly, then smiled again and turned to his right. "Deirdre, nice to see you again. Have you been running? You look robust."

Deirdre giggled—a rare and strange sound for Patrick to hear. "Every day. It's been nice, being back at Patrick's apartment." She stood up as Aamir walked to her and embraced her warmly.

"You're a saint, Deirdre. Staying all this time. A saint. He's lucky."

"No, I'm not. I'm really not."

"Well, it's rarer than you think. Rarer than you'd like to know."

He turned again and walked back towards the door. "I've got to get in to a couple other rooms. But I hope Doctor Shin will have some news for you later. I'll stop by afterwards, if it's OK. Check up on you. Tell me to go away if you're not in the mood."

"Thanks, Aamir. It's really good to see you—well, such as I can." He smiled, shifting his attention for a moment to the blobs of dark absence that dotted his visual field: he tricked his eyes around them, tracing the room and Aamir's place within it.

Aamir laughed, gave a small wave, and was gone.

They sat then in silence, Patrick and his mother, wondering separately how strange it was, this disproportionate arrangement: most of the doctors were so disabled when it came to affection—or, really, human connection full-stop. And at the other end of the economic spectrum, holding so little power, most of the nurses seemed to understand their charges as part of a large extended family: not precisely loving to everyone who came through those doors, but compassionate to a fault, as if they knew by both intuition and trade that while they could not *like* everyone equally, they *could* equally *care*. How bizarre that an institution developed over the centuries to foster and promote healing—to *enact* it—could be so defined by disequilibrium when it comes to simple kindness. How tragic, how bungled, how flawed.

Patrick thought of these things and wondered at their place in the flow of things, marveled at their stupidity. Deirdre wasn't surprised: in the long tail of history, after all, nurses had usually been women and doctors had usually been men. "Men screw everything up, to their own advantage," she thought, then added, "when women screw up, we *all* lose."

Interlude

They struck us as lovely, both the word and the object it described: Lace. What a perfect way to characterize the way we'd made room for ourselves, created space. Of course we had no sense of the view; it was, for all intents and purposes, an aerial photograph as seen by someone who is not, and has not ever been, able to fly.

The word summoned, for Patrick, distant memories of an old-age home, a place he'd visited often as a kid. He couldn't remember who'd lived there; but he knew that once a year, he and group of others were taken in to sing carols for whomever they were. The other kids were horrified by the place, moving through it methodically, on tip-toe, as if scared they'd set off a trap, as if worried they might trip a fuse. They shrank when the old people touched them or wanted a hug, drawing themselves up to become as small and invisible as possible.

Not Patrick. He'd loved those visits, looked forward to them even. He dressed up for them. And when it was time for singing, despite his not being a singer, he belted out the carols with such force that he carried the group, drew such focus that the small, aged audience didn't even notice that the other children were mostly just silently moving their mouths. And when he was called for a hug, he set himself forth with abandon, arms stretched out, squeezing hard.

We witnessed Patrick's remembering of that scene, paid attention. We understood it, appreciated its charisma. We even felt moved. We had gradually begun to feel for him by then, in the sense that we had a sense of him as a person, and in some vague, inchoate way, wished him well.

We had been decimated by the first round of hospital treatments, brought down to smaller numbers, left for dead. But we had not been obliterated completely, as they were beginning to understand. We were still at work—slowed down by the toll of surviving, but at work nonetheless.

And it was difficult work. Bone is called hard tissue for a reason. It is made, or has made itself, to withstand serious impact, major stress. It is not easy to get inside, to carve out a little path. It takes persistence, perseverance, and a healthy tolerance for drudgery. It takes time. Humans need drills to get through bone. We had only ourselves. Think about that.

Although he didn't quite know it yet, didn't recognize it for what it is, he was beginning to feel for us, too, to have a sense of us. He felt that we were there, knew that he was not alone. Not consciously. But he knew all the same.

It was during this period that we really began to pay attention, caught on to how storytelling summons others in to its swirl. We even tried to help him along, nudging a focus on specific parts by remembering them ourselves, collectively, in unison, lined up to the poles.

PART IV

25

"We may need to remove the leg."

Deep in a distant corner, Deirdre leaned back, her strong hands grasping empty air. She collapsed into a chair, bent down, and the floor was moving—spinning, like a circus or a mid-century tin toy, spinning to where she could no longer see it. Sheila came rushing with a plastic pan, ready to catch what she knew was coming. Deirdre had not been sick for nearly thirty years. But here, those words echoing in her ears, she vomited into the pan, her eyes now filled up with stars. And the doctor turned, unable to handle so much unmoored, and silently left the room.

Sheila watched, skeptical but not surprised, as the door closed behind him, just catching the tail of his coat. He seemed to struggle there on the other side, then quickly whisked the white fabric from where it was caught and rushed down the sterile hall. She had known many of these men in her twenty years as a nurse, and had developed that sophisticated sense of irony that complemented her own gestures of care with a quietly insubordinate smirk that said "I know what you are." She turned to Deirdre, who was now embarrassed by her untidy display. Deirdre wiped at the corners of her mouth, her eyes sunk defeatedly back, her skin flushed with the silent erotics of fear. Sheila turned to check Patrick, who—though he could not quite see her just now—seemed to know that his mother had faded somehow. "What happened?" he chirped from the bed, "Mom? What happened?"

Sheila turned back to Deirdre, who in the intervening seconds had recomposed herself, now smoothing the pleats of her pants with steady hands. "Nothing, Patrick," Deirdre said, "I just needed to sit down. I'm sure he'll be right back."

"What did he mean, 'remove the leg'?" Patrick asked.

"I don't know, son. He'll be right back. Everything's fine. Everything is going to be fine. Sheila, can you reach that book? The notebook. It's on the table."

Quick, like a hawk, Sheila passed the book to Deirdre and simultaneously felt for the IV tube laced droopily across the bed. "You've nearly pulled it out again. Lean back. Lean *back*, I'll check the plug."

Like a child at the site of a natural disaster, Patrick did as he was told—precisely, resigned to his minor role. Sheila worked like a watchmaker, pulling back the tape, checking the connection beneath, then re-covering it all in little more than a tick. She lifted Patrick's arm, then placed it—curated it, almost—delicately at his side. "*Child*. Can you please lie still for a moment. Like this. OK?"

He was looking at the opposite wall. He could sense her eyes on him, feel them pressing into his; and for the first time, in this moment that he knew was not at all about him, he realized that he could no longer participate fully in the usual meeting-of-eyes that humans hold so dear. "Look me in the eyes," he thought; "look me in the eyes. I will only ever *remember* what that means."

He remembered how Aamir, weeks before, had found a space to negotiate within Patrick's fractured field of vision, to line their visions up, as if he held secret knowledge of an even more secret retinal geography. He felt that this moment, here in this bed, was significant, what they call an *epiphany*, at the same time that he felt emptied out by its occurrence. He tried to straddle these modes of consciousness: on one hand, he wanted to weep, so taken aback he was by the insistence of the loss; but on the other hand, he felt astonished at the seriousness of this shift, thought of it as a rupture, wondered how he could learn from it and what it might mean.

But feeling won out: his eyes were suddenly soft and calm in that way that eyes are when they begin to fill with tears; they were soothed, as if held in a well-known embrace. In this moment weeping was more flow than eruption, more sigh than choke, more silk than wool. He lay still, as he had been told to do, and silent, as he knew he should, and so gave no indication to the others in the room that anything—anything more than they already knew—was wrong.

Sheila had gone to tend to Deirdre, and they sat locked up in urgent exchange, Sheila stroking Deirdre's arm, Deirdre grasping Sheila's leg. "You're all right," Sheila breathed. "You're all right; you know you're all right. Take a moment. You need to take a moment."

"But he," Deirdre began, then froze.

"He is fine. Look at me. You need to take a moment. You have been strong, you have held up. But your strength needs a rest. *They*," she spitted this word out, like a poison, while jerking her head back and across in the direction of the doctors' hall, "do not understand this. But I do. When *they* tell you to leave, they just want you out of the way. But when *I* tell you to go, it is because I know."

Deirdre, stoic and almost shy, nodded deliberately.

Sheila went on. "Now. You need to go out for a while. Walk down the street, turn left, then left again, and there's a small park. Go sit, or keep walking if you'd rather. Take twenty minutes. I will not leave this room." She turned briefly back to the bed, intending only to glimpse; but she caught a quick sign that Patrick had come undone—silently, without expression, which is to say in the worst possible way. She maneuvered quickly to block Deirdre's view as she lifted her out of the chair, turned her to the wall to steer her towards the room's door. Brilliantly, like a cryptographer, she framed this blocking so that Deirdre would not resist it: "I've got you. He can't see you with me here. Keep going. Just keep walking. Twenty minutes."

And Deirdre was gone, clutching the book like a shield.

Sheila paused for a moment at the door. She thought of her promise to herself, years ago, never to get entangled in the lives of white folks. She thought, as she often did, of Bobby (now so long gone), of the world they'd begun to build, closed to outsiders and richer than theirs, more full in its potential to structure social support on both small and large scales. She'd had to soften her stance somewhat when she took this job, had to reconcile herself to dystopia. And she'd found, over the years, that caring for all who came into this place did not mean that she cared any less passionately for the intense paradoxes of home—its pleasures and pains, its stumblings and strengths, its commingling of recognition and otherness. She resolved here, again, to do her job, to do it well. She allowed herself a space of thick compassion for these two—Patrick but mostly Deirdre, who was again glimpsing the possibility of losing a child, as Sheila had done so many years before—for the time that they were here. She even permitted herself to remember them; she authorized these eventual memories but did not grant them more detail than they deserved. She turned back to the room.

"Now as for you," she began gently then stopped short, seeing that he had dried his face and shut down. He seemed to stare passively at his feet, though she knew he could not see them. She detoured, acknowledging the turn: "So much your mother's child."

Though he had learned from Deirdre how to compose himself, his compositions were rarely complete. And so as he spoke, he began to shatter again—because he was not precisely sure about what he should be resilient, and so could not marshal the right form of self-possession. "I don't know what's happening. That man said something about removing the leg—whose leg, mine?—and then mom went quiet, which usually means she's either lost or upset, and now she's gone. And I think she saw me start to fall apart, which would only have made it worse for her."

"Your mother just went out for a walk. She'll be back."

"I know, I could hear you. I knew what you were doing." He paused, thinking more slowly now. "You're very good, you know. You may be the smartest person in this place."

"Sure I am. Now listen." Her voice hardened, but only to the point of urgency—not steel. "Your mother becomes steadier when she sees you begin to fall apart. And you, you do not want your mother to see you upset. An impasse."

Patrick was stunned, called out. "An impasse," he repeated back to her in admission.

"Yes. So let her see you cry. Let her watch you. Do not shore yourself up. You do not have to be brave. Everything doesn't have to be OK."

"I don't have to be brave."

"You don't have to be brave."

He looked in her direction, then down again, worrying the thin blanket with his right hand. There was a smudge near its edge, a stain where something had refused to be washed away, that he could just make out at the edge of his visual field. Following his gaze, Sheila looked at the spot, considered taking the blanket and bringing another; but she decided then to leave it, to leave him something to consider. She watched as he moved his eyes to the left, tracking the spot. He was learning, without knowing it, how to focus on something small, how to trace intricacy, how to find and fix the most minor constituent part of a larger whole.

"I don't have to be brave."

26

Deirdre again walked the halls. They had become so familiar to her that she could have walked them in her sleep: here the nurses' station, blocked off from the clean linoleum floors with a barricaded desk, stacked high with files and forms. Upstairs the wide glass rooms, left open to peering passers-by, keeping at bay some of the most severe cases; inside lay bodies, all trussed up, wired to the walls and to mobile machines that flickered and moaned. Behind her the cordoned-off doctors' offices, safe with their closed doors, their sanctuaries more pristine than anywhere else. She came to the stairwell and elevator bank and, choosing to walk rather than ride, pulled open the heavy door and began to descend. One foot in front of the other. She ignored the handrail, hugging the notebook close, steadying herself with sheer resolve. One foot in front of the other, each step a near-disaster. These were heavy stairs, deep and wise. They had felt the tread of many before her, and would continue their work long after she was gone. One foot in front of the other, she turned slowly at the landing and continued on. Here were posters, all function no design: emergency exit, in case of fire, no exit from level 2. They flashed at the edge of her vision, urging her on, one foot in front of the other. She reached the ground floor.

Standing just inside the door, Deirdre could see through the slender window there a wider, open hall. A cluster of chairs to the right welcomed visitors and guests, urging their forgiveness for the inevitable long wait. To the left, a small reception desk, a lamp, a potted plant. She watched as a group of men in blue scrubs rushed past, ignoring those waiting in the chairs. But the people sitting there all stared expectantly at the quickly moving tribe: like a choreographed troupe, or synchronized swimmers, or an audience at Wimbledon, they turned their heads in unison, the disappointment of "no new information" settling in collectively. They sighed together, then looked back at the magazines and newspapers draped forlornly across their laps. She watched as a gurney was rolled across the room, empty but for a tangle of blankets and a single, small pillow that was still bent with the impression of someone's head. She watched as a name was called and a single, eager woman stood up from her chair and walked quickly to the desk. She opened the door, catching her first full breath of sweet scented air as she stepped out of the stairwell and into the lobby. It smelled like a lie (told earnestly and with good intent—but a lie all the same).

She crossed the room quickly, trying not to glance in anyone's direction, and was through the large front doors within seconds. Now outdoors, she passed the smokers huddled together and watching her guiltily. She passed the newspaper boxes. She passed the ambulance gate. One foot in front of the other, she followed Sheila's directions without thinking much about them, walking as if on a mission. Deirdre turned left, then left again.

The park wasn't much, but it was set back from the street and, more importantly, was presently empty. She crossed to a bench resting in the light of a streetlamp, checked it was dry, and sat down. Her eyes softened, relaxing their attention into the middle-distance as she sank back into the bench.

Time passed, and passed again.

The sound of scattering leaves jarred Deirdre from her silence. She turned just in time to see them gather in a heap then pop apart again as a breeze rushed through, spreading them across the walk. One of the leaves, bright yellow at the center but crusted with brown at its edge, seemed to float towards her, stopping just at the edge of her shoe. She watched it tremble as it touched her, settle down, then skitter off into the grass. She looked down at her lap, where the notebook—now quarter-filled with jargon and math—lay closed and still. Its cover was clean and blank, but signs of wear had begun to express themselves at its corners. She opened the book, turning to the first page with room, and pulled a pen out of her pocket.

In the upper-right corner, Deirdre wrote "29 December" and underlined it twice. Then, above the first line: "Dr Shin"; she hesitated there, seeming to summon some kind of will, then continued. "Dr Shin: moth-eaten bone."

She paused again, watching the words as if they would move.

"Also called fir-tree or sun-burst."

And then, almost in spite of herself, she picked up the pace, writing quickly and evenly across the page, but with an increasing sense of urgency, out of control.

What she wrote was not for others' eyes, and she was vaguely aware that she should have begun on a new page, which could be torn out and hidden away later on. But she bypassed this concern, not willing or able to stop the flow.

She considered, in writing, the strange beauty of metaphor: moth-eaten, like lace; fir-tree, evoking snow and gifts and (best of all) the chocolate-covered cherries her family always ate; sun-bursts at the beach, in the form of urchins and anemones and, in minimalist mode, the fragile sand dollars she used to collect. She considered how metaphor works like a salve, softening the sting of diagnostic description; she wondered, what is this function, and where did it come from, and why use beauty as an antidote to fear? She tried to imagine other ways to explain the action of disintegrating bone: melting, evaporating, crumbling; "bone erodes," she wrote, "washed away like a beach"; she briefly conceived of bone as architecture, as the hidden beams and screws that lay out and limit a space. She wrote the word itself, "bone," seventeen different ways, stretching the boundaries of her handwriting to make it look other unto itself. She wrote it backwards then, and upside down, concentrating so as to get the letters right. She tried to think of synonyms for "bone" and, finding none, listed out words then conjoined it with something else. Bone-dry. Bone china. Bone meal.

After the last, she felt a sudden shot of memory: years and years ago, early in the marriage with Jonathan. A small limestone house in a wide open space, suffocating in its intimacy. One of the few times Jonathan cooked: a fish-fry, mashed potatoes, peas. Patrick was young, but unusually linguistic; while most kids his age spoke in sentences, he seemed to create paragraphs on the fly. They were sitting at the table, and Patrick was describing a bright red fire-engine toy as if it were an object of astonishing beauty. They had noticed how strange his play was: rather than pushing the toy around, he would only clean it, polishing the sides and top with a rag, scraping out the grooves in its tires, washing its plastic windshield. Suddenly, in that moment at supper, she had become aware that he had stopped speaking, uncharacteristically cut off halfway through a word. His eyes had grown huge, and he seemed frozen in anticipation; but he was not smiling, his mouth instead shaped into a wide, round O. He made a strange sound then, between a cough and a laugh.

With uncharacteristic grace, Jonathan had leapt from his chair, lifting his son up and back to clear space. Deirdre had sat blankly and watched, too stunned by Jonathan's move to move herself. "A bone," Jonathan said, "in his throat. He has a fishbone in his throat." In action now, Jonathan had deftly stood Patrick up, saying, "Stay calm, son. Breathe through your nose. Think about your truck" as he quickly jogged to the kitchen for the phone. Still frozen with surprise, Deirdre watched this scene as if it were happening on a stage: Patrick standing, staring wildly back at her as he tried to focus on his breath, Jonathan diligent and quick in looking up the number and calling the clinic.

It had all been fine, in the end. A quick trip to have a doctor (bow-tie, speckled shirt, soothing voice, over-large hands) reach with a tool down Patrick's throat to extract the bone; Patrick panting and gracious when it was done, staring with rare awe at his father; a gift from the nurse of a toy, for being such a brave boy; and all the while, Deirdre moving slowly, a minor player, doing what she was told. It had all been fine.

Deirdre lifted her head and looked at the sky, best she could with the lamp shining down. It was dark now, fully night. Through the haze of the city's gleam, she could just make out a few dozen stars, gathered together in congress high above the horizon. She looked down at her feet, placed by sheer chance in the very center of a patch where the grass had worn away from all of those who had sat here before. She looked straight ahead, saw the brick facade of an old building staring back at her across the small park. It was quicksand, this, all of it, dragging her down and holding her under; she could not get a grasp of its edges, couldn't push or pull her way out.

And then she grew angry, truly angry. The nerve of that man, talking about her son's leg as if it were just a thing—a thing to be discussed in casual chatter like it meant nothing. The veins in her hands started to pulse with new energy, drumming with indignation. *The nerve.* She briefly concocted a wish: before being licensed, doctors should have to become sick, laid up in the hospital with no means to leave. Give them smallpox, or a very bad flu. They should learn what it feels like, having your body talked about in such object-driven ways. She settled herself into her anger for a few moments, sat with it.

And then she stood up, checked the bench to ensure she didn't leave anything behind, and walked back.

27

"I'm sorry I left the room." Doctor Shin sat now in a chair, elbows balanced on his knees, looking unkempt. "The truth is, I was shocked by what I saw in those X-rays. I called in a few colleagues to talk about them, make sure I wasn't off-base. As I told you before, the infection has spread. It's all over the place, inside the bone. It has taken over. The upper third of the bone is completely moth-eaten."

"We understand," Deirdre said. "The question is, what do we do?"

"He'll need surgery. As soon as possible. But I can't do it."

"What do you mean, you can't do it? You told us you could."

"I don't think I can. Look," he looked at his feet, "we're not really trained to say we can't do things in our specialty. I'm not pulling your leg—I mean, I'm not *lying* to you or just trying to get out of something. This is a very complicated problem. The left femur is riddled with bacteria, it's enormously fragile. That explains the pain. I don't know how you've been up at all, Patrick, without shattering that bone. And I just don't think I'm the right guy for the surgery. I've never done anything like this. You need someone with a depth of experience in this kind of work."

"Do you know anyone?" Deirdre asked.

"I've already started making calls. There are two guys in San Francisco who are experts in severe osteomyelitis. I've called them. There's an entire unit down in Palo Alto, I've called them too. None of them have beds available right now."

"So what do we do?"

"I'll discharge you tonight. Maybe they haven't even finished with all your check-in paperwork—anyway, I'll discharge you tonight. Go home, and be very careful on that leg. We'll get you the first available bed, call you, tell you where to go."

"How long?" Deirdre asked.

"Could be a couple days, maybe a little longer. You'll be top of the list."

They looked at each other. For the first time since Doctor Shin had returned, Patrick spoke to him: "Tell you what. I've got a different plan. I refuse."

"Patrick," Deirdre said sharply. "Patrick."

"No, mom, listen." He turned back to the doctor. "Write this down, or whatever you need to do. I *refuse* to be discharged. Whatever I'm supposed to do or sign to enable you to discharge me without liability, I refuse. I will not leave this room, not until you figure out where I'm going next, and send me there."

"Well," Doctor Shin said, sitting up, shocked by this turn, "well, Patrick, I mean, we're not a *hotel*." He spread his arms out widely, gesturing to the walls. "We need this room for others, you know, others who are in a similar boat. Think of them."

"Look, doctor. I appreciate your honesty tonight. I really do. Thank you for saying you are not qualified. I get what guts that took. Thank you. But, please, do not play my sympathies for others who need help. Do not play me. You've just told me that my leg should have shattered. I will not now get up and go home, waiting for someone to call saying something's opened up somewhere. Forget it. You've just told me my bone is filled up with infection. I'm not taking that home. I refuse." He looked—neither kindly nor unkindly—at Doctor Shin, nodded. "You need this bed for someone else. So go find me a place where they can help me. Please."

Twenty minutes later, Sheila—newly invested with sharp and sass-filled energy—was tidying up the sheets on Patrick's bed. "Oooh—*child*. You got the whole ward talking tonight. Everybody! Never seen anything like that. Never." She snapped the sheets up, fluffing them out and then tucking them back in. "Told that doctor what's what. You got *all* the nurses talking tonight!"

"I couldn't just leave," Patrick said, "not after what he told me. I mean—"

"Oh, I know. I know. Did exactly what you should've done. But I have *never* seen someone so sick in bed tell a doctor he wasn't leaving. 'I refuse,' you said. 'I *refuse*.' Tell him!" She cocked her hip to the side as she finished the bed, patting it with her hands to smooth it out. "Oooh. I think I'm gonna make it through my night shift now. That gave me a *bump*."

Patrick gave her a half-smile. He was not proud of himself, couldn't summon any sense of ownership over what had just happened. But he did feel gratified, like he had seized something like power and used it towards the good. "We'll see how long it lasts. Maybe he'll send the cops."

"Oh, you're not going anywhere. Don't you worry about that. Not until we get you that transfer. I've got your back. And there's an army of nurses out there, won't let anybody get within ten feet of you. Don't you worry about that." She went out, laughing as she walked down the hall. "I *refuse*!" he heard her say again.

Deirdre watched this scene from her chair. Her son's outburst, his standing his ground, had assuaged something in her, a worry that he had given up or given over his sense of himself and his needs. She watched him now as he lay quietly, eyes closed, breathing slowly, deliberately. He was her son, no doubt about that. She got up and walked to his bed, where she began stroking his hair. She leaned in to him, down to his ear. "I am so proud of you," she whispered. "I am so proud."

It was after midnight now. Patrick and Deirdre were both sleeping, Patrick in his bed, tucked tight, Deirdre curled up on the recliner she'd found down the hall. Because she was so small, she fit neatly in tidy spaces, nestled in. Sheila poked her head in occasionally, checking in but trying not to disturb their sleep. Every few hours, she had to rouse Patrick to take his vitals. He would stir, hover just above the precipice of consciousness, and then drop right back off. Unusual for her, Deirdre didn't awake during any of these intermittent visits: she slept straight through. The night passed easily and without demonstration.

When Patrick finally, fully awoke, it had nearly gone eight o'clock, the latest he had slept naturally in a very long time. Doctors had finished their rounds; in a tense and quite moving scene, Deirdre had insisted that they skip Patrick for now, his rest being more important than an official check-in, given that everyone knew they were just waiting for him to be moved. There was no need to rouse him, no point. "Just move along," she had said, blocking the door with her tiny frame. "Thank you, doctor, yes, we know. It's protocol. But he has not slept in so long, I really think it's more important he get on with it. Look here," pointing at the chart, "Sheila took his vitals an hour ago. All normal, all good. Please. We'll call you when he wakes up."

Doctor Pettle had arrived just then; and since it was easier for the hospitalist on duty to yield to another doctor—to yield to another man—he moved on, just as Deirdre had asked, with a professional nod and: "Good. *You're* with him. Check in with you later, Doctor."

Deirdre fumed, but hid the fumes.

Now Patrick was beginning to sit up; Sheila had brought him a small breakfast as she was getting ready to leave. He was looking at it carefully, sitting there on the tray. He was wondering what was underneath the plastic cloche: had she said eggs? Pancakes? He couldn't remember. He hoped there was meat.

"I think," Doctor Pettle said, eyeing him closely, "that one of the most important turning-points in all of this happened last night."

Patrick looked at him. "You mean the X-ray?"

"No. If I had been here, I would have told them they could not discharge you. The fact that *you* took on that role, standing your ground.... Well, Patrick, I know you're facing a lot of unknowns right now, and they must be frightening. But you have to know how important that was. *You* took that role. You stood your ground. And you made the correct decision, against the will of the surgeon in the room. That's remarkable."

Patrick shrugged. "I just didn't want to go home, not knowing there'd be another long wait, another check-in." He lifted the cover. It was eggs, and there was sausage. He faintly smiled. "I just didn't want to go home." He pulled the tray closer to him, picked up a fork.

"Well, you did absolutely the right thing. Absolutely. And let me also say," he turned to Deirdre, "how grateful we must be to Doctor Shin. That kind of honesty—it is rare. I don't want to think what might have happened if his ego had gotten in the way, if he'd decided to go ahead with a surgery he was not prepared to perform."

"I guess so," Deirdre said. "I guess so."

"Really, Deirdre, we should be enormously thankful. That simple moment of clarity on his part, of egoless honesty, very well might have saved Patrick's life."

"Again," Patrick said. Doctor Pettle turned back to him. "Saved my life *again*. I guess I owe a lot of gratitude." He was eating his eggs. A tiny bit of yellow was stuck to the outside of his lower lip.

"Yes," Doctor Pettle said. "As we all do." He looked at his lap, momentarily fogged in a thought. "As we all do."

Sheila came in to say goodbye. She would be back later that day, she told them: another night shift. "You keep refusing," she told Patrick, and then quickly turned to leave.

28

Sheila decided to walk.

Most days she took the bus, but today she felt like traveling alone. She pulled the straps of her bag tight against her shoulder and turned left on Telegraph; her favorite house in the area—large, sky blue—sat bashfully across the street. She paid it little mind this morning, focused instead on the road in front of her. It would take her over an hour to walk home, more if she circled around the lake. The bus would have taken twenty-seven minutes door-to-door; but she wanted time to think.

She watched her feet fall, one in front of the other, on the still-damp sidewalk. She passed Woolsey before she really got going—not speedy, but warmed from the hike. She was thinking of Bobby. He was seven years old the day he woke up with what seemed like a flu, stiff joints, aching all over. She remembered the date exactly: December 15, 1974. Two days after Betty disappeared. It was foggy; it had rained briefly the day before. He hadn't woken up like usual. She'd had to go in and coax him out, pull his blankets over and off. And still he lay there, his arms out flat to his sides, his legs crooked up like a tent. "Bobby," she had said, "I don't have *time* for this today. Bobby, baby, get *up*." His eyes were wide open, watching the ceiling.

"Mama, I don't feel right."

This time next year, it would be thirty years gone since that day. Hard to believe, she thought, crossing against the light at Alcatraz—hard to believe he'd be in his thirties now, a full-grown man with a life of his own. Hard to believe, hard to think about what he might have done. She'd called the Community School that day, told them not to expect him. "Sick in bed," she'd said, "I'm keeping him home."

"Meningitis," the doctor had told her when she finally took him in, a week later. She'd assumed it was a flu. But he'd had some small seizures, and the local folks didn't know what to do. She'd taken him in, and the doctor said, "How long has he been like this?"

"Week or so. Thought it was the flu."

The doctor looked regretfully but also critically at Sheila: "Should have brought him sooner. Let's see what we can do." Did she detect something else in his eyes? Disapproval? Distaste? Nothing new there; young mother, mid-twenties, not poor but not rich either. Bobby was dead within the month.

She was making good time: into the fifties now, coming up to the overpass. She considered crossing west, down to MLK, gave it a good half-thought but continued on her way. One foot in front of the other, she passed a liquor store, not giving it a second glance. She passed the hospital's physical therapy and rehab center, set so far south from the main campus. In the parking lot, she watched as an old black man, done up in Sunday best, worked to get into his car. His daughter was nearby, or maybe just a friend; she steadied his walker as he lowered himself, arms shaking, into the passenger seat. He was wearing a bright red bow-tie, tight at his neck, and sharp black tweed. Finally down, he looked up and caught Sheila's eye. She gave him a smile, and he nodded in return, lips tight and proud.

"You good, Daddy? Let's get your legs in," his daughter said, moving the walker out of the way. "There we go, nice and easy. Easy as pie. Good?" She stood up, folded the walker, and went to put it in the back. Sheila watched as the woman took a moment, hands on the trunk; she looked at the sky, breathed deeply, then shook her head and looked down. Finally she brushed off her pants in the front, pulled the keys from the trunk's lock, and walked to the driver's side.

"One foot in front of the other," Sheila thought, "in whatever time it takes. Not much more you can do than that." She walked under the highway as cars whisked by on their way to Orinda; she picked up her pace, thinking through what was waiting for her at home. She walked in silence amidst the city noise, which she did not mind.

Back in the room, Patrick was sitting up, watching as Doctor Pettle flipped through those images once again, holding them up to the light. Tugboat Tim had come and gone; he'd asked if he could stay the night, give Deirdre a break, but she had once again refused. He would get back as soon as he could, he'd told them—but it might be a while, maybe not until after the exercise with the failed ship. But even so, he'd be on-call for them; should anything happen, should they need anything, early morning, middle of the night, whenever, just call. Patrick watched as he and Deirdre embraced—warmly, as if he were one of her own sons.

"Yeah, wow, look at that. How *have* you been walking?" Doctor Pettle looked faintly astonished.

"I wouldn't call it *walking*, exactly."

"How have you been up at *all*?"

Patrick shrugged unseen.

Doctor Pettle put the images down on his lap, removed his glasses, rubbed the bridge of his nose again.

"Do you have a sense of what they want to do? The surgery, I mean."

Doctor Pettle kept his glasses off, cocked his eyebrows. "It's hard to say. I don't think Doctor Shin *knows* for sure, which is part of why he's sending you to someone else." He looked over at Patrick. "If I had to guess, I'd say they'll try the least invasive option first. Depends on how urgent they think things are. First stage would probably be—let's see, I'm guessing they'd try to impregnate the bone with antibiotic beads." There was a pause as Doctor Pettle looked up at the ceiling, doing some silent computations. Patrick stared towards him, stunned.

"I'm sorry, but you're going to have to say that again."

Doctor Pettle snapped to attention, looked over at him, then put his glasses back on. "What's that?"

"What did you just say? *Impregnate* my bone?"

"Oh—yes, right. That *does* sound strange, doesn't it?" He smiled. "Funny, the kind of language one gets accustomed to. OK, so the problem is that the IV antibiotics you've been taking have not been able to penetrate the affected bone well enough to treat the infection. Right?"

"Right."

"So they need to get antibiotics into the bone. Yes?"

"OK, yes."

"And if they can't do that directly through the bloodstream, they certainly would not be able to do it with pills that you swallow. So the next option is to get them in manually: literally, to place them inside the bone in such a way that they will be effective for days or even weeks at a time. Like a slow-release pill, but physically inside your bone."

"Got it. How do they do that?"

"They imbed the antibiotics in little beads made of a special cement, then open you up, drill into the bone, and place the beads into your bone by hand."

"Oh my God," Patrick said after a moment. "And they just leave them there?"

"Well, no, they do have to go back and remove them eventually. They link them all together with suture thread, like a string of pearls. Makes it easier to get them back out. In severe cases, I believe they repeat the process several times." He thought. "I think they've begun developing biodegradable options that don't need to be removed. I'm not sure where those options stand, whether they're in use clinically."

Patrick felt faint, but he did not give in to this feeling. "OK, so that's the first step. What if that doesn't work?"

"So that's where things get complicated. Are you sure you'd like to talk about this? We could wait, see what the surgeon eventually says."

"I'd rather know now what's possible. I'm fine, really. Lay it on me." It is worth noting that Deirdre was not in the room, as she would certainly *not* have encouraged this conversation.

"OK. So. If they decide that there's too much necrosis—if the bone is already too dead, or too much of it, to risk waiting, then they'll need to debride the dead parts, cut them away and remove them. What happens next depends on how much they remove. Let's say they take the entire upper part of the femur—the ball of your hip—then they'll need to replace it with a prosthetic. But that's risky; bacteria are attracted to the materials used to make prostheses, so it's important to ensure the infection is *completely treated* before placing an implant."

"So, what, I'd be without a hip for a while? Leg just dangling there?"

Doctor Pettle smiled. "Imagine *that*! No, not exactly. Once they removed the dead part of the bone, they'd use it to make—in the operating room, mind you, while you're lying there—a cement model of it, which, like the beads, they would fill with antibiotics and then implant in place of the hip. And later, they'd replace *that* with an actual prosthetic."

Patrick thought about this, did some computations of his own. "This is going to be a long process."

"Most certainly, Patrick. Most certainly. You have quite a road ahead of you. I hope you trust that you do not walk it alone."

Patrick smirked, "Well actually, I do not walk it at *all*."

Doctor Pettle let forth one of his little laughs. "I love that you can make jokes. I absolutely love that."

"Better than the alternative."

"Yes. More healing than the alternative, too, laughter being medicine and all."

Just then, Deirdre returned. "What's going on in here?" she asked smilingly.

"Oh, nothing," Patrick said. "Just chatting. Is it nice outside?"

"It's chilly, not too bad."

"Do I know who my nurse is yet?"

"I don't think they've been able to assign you one. Apparently someone called in sick, messed up the orders. Seven beds to a nurse on this floor, so they're trying to figure out what to do."

"Is Aamir still here?"

"I haven't seen him. He probably left around the same time as Sheila."

Patrick reached for the button and pushed it. Within moments he felt the slow release, the slight shift in his muscular temperament, the physical exhale.

29

"Good news," said Doctor Shin. "We've found you a bed."

Deirdre shot up from her chair. "You're kidding. So fast?"

"I pulled some strings, got you a spot in the city. We'll transfer you tonight, get you there in an ambulance, have you all set up to meet the surgeon tomorrow morning. They might want to take some of their own images when you get there, so you should prepare yourself for a long night."

"What strings," Patrick thought, "what strings did he need to pull? And who was displaced?" He didn't dare ask this out loud.

"Patrick, I am so sorry for what you are going through. I'm sorry that I couldn't help you more. I'll keep an eye on you from here, keep in touch with Doctor Pettle. Stay with it, OK? You can make it through this. Stay with it."

"I will. Thank you for bringing me back in and, now, for getting me a bed."

"I'm just sorry it's all happened the way it has. Not to speak out of turn—I wasn't on the case before and don't know all the ins and outs—but you should never have been discharged the first time."

"Well, we are where we are. Nothing to do about it now."

"No. I suppose not. Well. I'll be off now. I've already signed the transfer paperwork. They'll be by to get you in a while."

It was nearing five o'clock, and the light outside was almost gone. Patrick felt a surge of anticipation again, excitement even. Things were happening; it was all progressing as it needed to progress. A step further than he was before. He was ready to go.

Within ten minutes of Doctor Shin's leaving, Deirdre had finished packing all of their things. She stood at the door, looking out into the hall. She walked back to the window, looked out at the street below, stayed there for a minute or so, then walked back to the door. She continued with this staccato pacing for more than half an hour before she finally sat down. "Where are they?" she asked the room.

It was two hours before they finally showed, two young paramedics with a nurse. First they went through his file, which had been photocopied for them to take with him; then took his vitals, ensuring he was safe to transport; then roughly moved him over to the orange gurney with collapsible legs. They rolled him away, the two paramedics, chattering among themselves as Deirdre followed with the bags. She was to drive Patrick's car, get there when she could. The ambulance's lights and sirens would be on, and she could not caravan behind them. They had drawn her a map of how to get there; she did not fully understand it, and she was worried about driving across the bridge and into the city. She did not tell them this.

"Kind of exciting," Patrick said to them in the elevator. "Riding in an ambulance with its lights on."

"Sure," one of the paramedics said.

"People pulling over to the side of the road, just for me. Kind of exciting."

"Sure," the guy said, "sure."

And it *was* exciting, for the first few minutes, before an intensity of disorientation overtook him. The sirens were on and the van kept moving, rare for a trip across the bridge. But lights flashed and trailed through the windows, stretching out across the interior, where he lay pinioned to the gurney—not actually tied down, but frozen with the sensation of being moved at high speeds. The lights from outside seemed not like what they were, but instead like what you might see on the walls of a late-night club, near the dance floor: whirling flashes and trails like the colored beams refracted endlessly by the surface of a disco ball.

When they arrived, he was pulled up and out of the ambulance, paramedics working and talking as if barely aware he was there at all. They took him through the emergency entrance to the main desk, where they were directed to leave him in the hall for a moment. "We've got other calls," the driver said. "Can't we just check him in?"

"Not now," the nurse on duty said sharply, "just wait." She turned and was gone, answering a telephone and chirping orders to another nurse in the same breath. Deirdre was nowhere in sight.

They wheeled him about fifteen feet away, parked him next to the wall in a busy hall. From there, he could see the squares of the ceiling, some emergency flood lights, and the tops of various signs hanging around the place. The meds had worn off; he was in pain.

"Guys," he said, "can you let them know my pain is out of control? Explain that I was just transferred, they had me on a drip at the other place and regular meds. Can you let them know? It's getting really bad."

"Nothing we can do," one of the paramedics replied. "Gotta wait 'til they're ready for you."

Two doctors whooshed past, white coats brushing up against the arms of the gurney. They were talking intently, ignoring everything else around them. Someone on a similar gurney had been left across from the automated doors where he'd been rolled in; that person seemed to be moaning now, not too loud, but urgently. There was no way for him to tell how much time was passing. His hip and leg throbbed, as if threatening to explode from the inside out. It was now a wet pain, like acidic candle wax, melting. "Is my mom here yet?"

The other man looked down at him. "Haven't seen her, but she'll have to go through the front entrance."

"Does she know what room I'm going to?"

"*We* don't even know what room you're going to."

The nurse called the man over; he disappeared, time passed, and then he returned. "Gave her his name, but she says she has no record. I gave her the transfer, she said she'll make a call."

More time, spreading out like magma across the room. Patrick began to count the holes in the ceiling tiles, starting at the lower left quadrant of one of them and counting across. He intended then to count up and do the simple math, but he kept losing his place in the tile, having to start over. This happened seven or eight times before the nurse suddenly appeared.

"Found him. Problem is we had a crash victim come in since the orders were written. She took the open bed in the orthopedic ward. So now we're full again." Patrick hadn't said anything, or made any kind of noise, but now his silence expanded: he withdrew into himself and tried to look away.

"So I've got him a bed up in the psych ward. It's not ideal, but it'll do. I've paged Doctor Mizrahi to let him know. He's in surgery now. He might be able to meet you up there later. More likely he'll come in the morning."

She handed the men a stack of papers and disappeared again. They put the pages on the gurney, on Patrick's chest, asked him to make sure they didn't fall, and began pushing him down the hall. An abundance of noise: footsteps constantly, arranged at differing paces; whispered mumblings between people walking together; and the near-constant sound of people moaning. Patrick tried to stare straight ahead—which, from his vantage, meant staring at those tiles— but he caught several faces in the blur as he was pushed. Some didn't seem to notice him; others caught him in their glare, but quickly looked away. Faces of all kinds in this place, all of them rushed or rushing, all of them tensed up with the urgency of their current directive, all of them infallible somehow in their verticality. He tried not to notice, but he could not help himself: they were all so obviously relieved not to be sick.

Deirdre had had a harrowing journey from the East Bay, and was anxious and exhausted from the drive. She had gotten lost twice, unable to see the map clearly as she drove; with no one to help navigate, she was left being both the teller and the told. On the verge of angry tears, she stood at the front desk of the hospital, gripping its edges, readying herself to leap over it, grab the keyboard, and find the record herself.

"Ma'am, I'm telling you, there's no record. Are you sure he was brought to *this* hospital?"

"He was transferred. As I said. Here."

"Well he must not be here yet, because he is *not* in the system."

"The doctor's name is Mizrahi. Can you please call him? He should know."

"Oh—wait a minute. Looks like they just got him in. You said he's on the orthopedic ward?"

"That's right."

"No, Ma'am, looks like somebody lied to you. He's up in psych."

"Excuse me?"

"He's going to psych. Probably on his way there right now. They just checked him in."

"What is '*psych*'?"

The woman at the desk looked at Deirdre, stood up, leaned in to her, and whispered: "Psychiatric ward. For psychiatric patients. You know, head trouble."

"But that's not why he's here."

"Well, sometimes when we're full ..."

"Are you telling me they're putting him in a mental hospital? An insane asylum?"

"Well, first of all, Ma'am," the woman said, sitting again, "we don't call it that anymore. It's the psych ward. And yes, that's where he's going."

"Thank you for your help."

Deirdre turned, grabbed the bags, and ran for the elevator.

In a different lift, from a different floor, Patrick was staring at the fluorescent bulbs above him as the metal cage grunted and shuddered in its shaft. Its speed was unreadable; it was either moving too fast or too slowly, but Patrick couldn't tell which. He'd always hated elevators, mistrusted their physics, getting in and getting out as quickly and efficiently as he could. This one seemed to be stopping on every floor, jerking to a halt without even the pretense of deceleration. Each time the doors opened, a group of people got off and got on, too many for the size of it. "One nice thing about being on a gurney," Patrick said to anyone listening, "is that nobody's going to crowd me." No one responded. He began breathing deeply, pacing himself.

When they'd finally arrived at his floor, the paramedics shoved the gurney out into a hall that seemed narrower and darker than the one below. There were gates at one side, a large orderly sitting and guarding them. Patrick sighed as they turned in the opposite direction and found the nurses' station.

Things were quieter here than where he had been brought in, but he could still hear echoes from that farther hall: more moaning, some yelps, someone shouting. The nurse on duty was a brisk, meticulous woman who had clearly been waiting for them. "Patrick, you made it," she said directly to him. "You'll be in the first room on the right, just over there. Sorry we've had to put you up here, but you'll be fine. We've got our eye on you."

The paramedics wheeled him in, moved him efficiently over to the bed, took the papers from him, and left. "Good luck," one of them said as they went.

It was a small but private room; as Patrick was learning, one of the benefits of hosting us was that he was never expected to share space. Now that he'd been properly diagnosed, he was quarantined from other patients, so fearful of our spread they all were. He looked from wall to wall, found the small window (barred, like everything else in this place seemed to be), saw that one of the ceiling lamps was out. The television perched on the wall was old and small. Everything smelled as if it had only just been cleaned. He thought for a moment of his room in the last place, how palatial it seemed next to this. And then he willed himself to forget it, to lose the comparison. It wasn't worth it.

His leg had caught fire, molten lava running inside the bone; it ebbed and flowed with the bubbling heat, stripping away tiny layer after layer as it rolled. He found the call button and pushed it, then closed his eyes and focused on breathing. In, hold, out, hold. Again and again. He thought of nothing else but his breath, or tried to. It was saturated with anxiety, this place, and lostness, and grief. They flanked him now, and even as he tried to ignore them he could feel them fingering his shoulders and sides, drawing him in.

30

The main hospital in San Francisco was first built in 1857, the result of two intense city problems. First, as with many similar public administrations, the local government was out of compliance with a federal regulation from back in DC, to provide indigent care: medical attention for those who lived on the street, or nearly, and could not afford to seek private care on their own. And second, vastly more disturbing: given the massive influx of migrants to town, the relevant officials had previously determined that the relatively new San Francisco needed both a hospital and a jail; but they could not afford both. They chose the jail. More important to lock people up than to heal them.

A travesty, the demotion of health to second-fiddle, especially when the first chair is occupied by incarceration—a travesty that had left the city with too much illness and injury on its hands. And so, finally, in 1857, a new hospital was built, close to downtown. It lasted fifteen years, outgrowing its size with the sheer volume of people arriving from all directions. Its current site on Petrero was chosen for the relative balm of the area: more sun, less fog. The new building, two stories of wood, opened in 1872.

Somehow, a miracle they said, it survived the great quake of 1906. But then it was again too small, the city itself having become one large hospital for the injured, the dying, the dead. There were other hospitals then, but they had mostly collapsed or burned out. When plague struck the following year, plans for reconstruction, same site, were already underway. The new buildings, brick and plaster in an Italianate design, were opened in 1915. Fifty years later, more buildings still. And more after that.

Its halls steeped in suffering, San Francisco General is one of the most important public places around. Ward 5B was made famous when HIV struck, the first clinical site dedicated to tracking and treating those who had been drawn into that viral flow. Its emergency departments, dubbed Level 1 Trauma, have served an expansive population, and have functioned as training grounds for not one but two of the most prestigious medical schools in the world. Its psychiatric wards are legendary.

Patrick found himself there now, mostly unaware of the distinctive import of the place. To him it recalled the Victorians, but fallen into disrepair. It seemed to cling to its sense of importance, of efficiency, of modest moralism—help all who need it—even as its sense of success, its ability to stay on top of things, lay just out of reach. Running to stand still, it made it through—but barely, and just in the nick of time.

It had taken an hour for a nurse to come in and hook him up to the drip. When she first arrived, Deirdre went off and came back again, trying to find someone in charge. But they were always away, tending to someone else, leaving her to confront the futility of good intentions. When someone finally came, she was visibly tired and overworked: "Name's Monique," she said. "I'm moving as fast as I can. This should get you going"—this in reference to the meds she pushed into his line manually, from a syringe—"I'll bring more every half-hour. Just 'til we get the patient-controlled machine, with the button, set up. Might take a while."

It was not, to put it bluntly, a happy arrival. It inspired no faith. But for now, as he drifted off into glassy calm, as the lava cooled, for now he was fine. Things were managed, only just. The pain had been overwhelming, flooding his body and brain so that nothing got through but it. When Deirdre had first arrived, he could not speak, frozen with it. She sat now by his bed. She stayed there, peering over at him, through the night. She did not leave, not once. She did not sleep.

There were thirteen beds to a nurse on this ward. So they rarely saw Monique that first night, never got to know her before she was replaced. In the morning it was someone else with his chart, taking his blood pressure and temperature. "I'm Ramón," he said while he pumped the cuff. "I'll be with you today."

Deirdre was writing in her book, keeping track as usual. Patrick asked, "Where am I? General? Last night was a haze."

"I heard. Yes, you're at General. Doctor Mizrahi is on his way up to see you now. Should be here soon."

"That's what they all say. 'Should be here soon.' Soon must mean something else in these places."

"We're very busy here," Ramón said. He did not speak again, finally finishing with his work and leaving briskly.

When Doctor Mizrahi arrived, he was orderly and neat, but obviously fresh from some long job—eyes focused, working through whatever else he had on his pile. "Patrick, hello. Sorry about these conditions. You should be downstairs, but we ran out of room."

"We heard," Deirdre said skeptically from her chair.

"You must be Patrick's mother," he said charmingly. "Hello. And thank you for spending so much time with him. I've heard you've been right beside him since this all started."

"I have."

"You must be exhausted, and very worried. So let's jump right into it. That OK with you, Patrick?"

"Yes. Please."

"As Doctor Shin told you, you have been through major septicemia: a bacterial infection that thrived in your bloodstream. In your first hospital stay, they treated most of the soft tissue. But they did not complete treatment of the bone. Your left femur, especially the top, in the hip, is still infected. We call this osteomyelitis. In your case, it's *chronic* osteomyelitis, which means that it's been there for a while."

"I take it you've read my file?"

"Every word. Twice."

Patrick had the feeling of familiarity: not like he had seen this man before, but as if the man had been paying attention to him, knew him thoroughly, from afar. He dropped whatever tension he had been holding, sank into the conversation. "Doctor Pettle explained what you'd probably want to do. Impregnate the bone with antibiotic beads."

"That's exactly right. I'll go in tomorrow morning, drill holes into the bone, and insert the beads."

"How long will they stay there?" Deirdre asked.

"About forty-eight hours, at which point I'll go in and replace them with fresh ones."

"Two surgeries, so close together?" Patrick asked. "Isn't that dangerous?"

"It's essential—and that's not the end of it. We'll probably do several more, depending on what I find when I get inside. I'd guess four total, over the next eight or nine days."

"*Four?*" Deirdre yowled from her chair. "*Four* surgeries?"

"That's my best guess. I'll know more after I've done the first." Doctor Mizrahi looked at her, then turned back to Patrick. "Does this all make sense to you?"

"Yes—but what if it doesn't work? What if the infection is still there?"

"Let's cross that bridge if we come to it, OK? Right now I want you to rest up. It's going to be an intense week." He paused, then turned carefully to Deirdre. "Would you mind if I have a few minutes alone with Patrick?"

"For what?" Deirdre asked without thinking, then quickly added: "I'm sorry. It's just that he keeps getting swept away from me. Yes, of course. I'll wait in the hall." She got up and walked out, closing the door behind her.

Doctor Mizrahi reached over, took Patrick's hand, placed it between his. He squeezed gently, applying just enough pressure to signify presence. He looked closely, so warmly, at Patrick. His eyes were deeply and vastly blue. "Now, Patrick, tell me how you are, how you really are. This can't be easy."

"It's not. I don't know, I guess I believe it'll all come out alright, one way or another. I just wish I could fast-forward through this part. Just skip it, get to the end."

"I wish I could make that happen. I really do."

"What if you just put me out for the next week? With anesthesia?"

Doctor Mizrahi smiled. "I think you'll understand that I can't. That would be very dangerous."

"I understand. I just wish...." He was cut short by a sudden swell of sad longing, "I just wish I could skip forward."

"Have you been feeling depressed?"

"I don't even know what that means in this context. How would that be different from feeling anything at all?"

"OK. I'm going to start you on another drug, one that will help with anxiety. If it starts to make you sink lower than you are now, if you start to feel even the slightest bit more sad or withdrawn, please have the nurse page me immediately. OK?" He squeezed Patrick's hand more firmly.

"OK."

"One more thing. Your surgery is tomorrow morning, 8 a.m. Before that, I want to take some images: some X-rays, maybe a CT scan."

"That's fine."

"I'd also like to do a spinal tap."

"A spinal tap? Why?"

"Just to make sure there's no infection in the fluid. The hip is so close to the spine. And I don't want to miss anything."

"When?"

"They'll do all of these today. Take you away to imaging, do the spinal tap here in your room."

"OK. So a busy day today, then surgery tomorrow."

"That's right. You up for it?"

"I'll do my best."

Doctor Mizrahi squeezed his hand more firmly still. "That's all I can ask. That's all anyone can ask."

Imaging went off without a hitch. Doctor Mizrahi had increased the pain meds allowance slightly and ordered a mild sedative. Patrick was wheeled from his room to the X-ray office in the basement, then down a long, narrowing hall to the CT machine. Both beds were cold once he was on them, like gunmetal benches in the middle of fall.

The spinal tap was more involved. A large, butch woman came into the room with a tray of tools. "Patrick? I'm Delilah."

"I've never met a Delilah!" he said from his bed. "Is that really your name?"

She smiled widely, mouth full of teeth. "It really is. You ready for our dance?"

"Is *that* what we're calling it?"

"Well, looks like I got a live one here. You must be feeling better than you were last night."

"Did I meet you last night?"

"Not really. We passed in the hall, when they were bringing you up. I gave you a wink. Thought you might have seen it, but I guess not."

Deirdre was asked to wait outside. There was a makeshift waiting room down the hall in an office no longer being used. Delilah began looking through a file she had brought with her; its tab was marked with a long, multi-colored sticker and anonymous numbers. "Yeah, you've been *through* it, you know." She shook her head as she read. "God I hate that they do this."

Patrick looked up. "Do what?"

"First sentence in your medical history includes the word homosexual. Why?" she asked the ceiling, "why in the world would they put that here?" She shook her head again. "Sorry. It's just, people like you and me haven't had the best luck with that kind of record-keeping."

"I had no idea that was in there."

"Of course not. Another reason to be furious." She was readying her tools as she spoke, arranging them on the tray. "People aren't even involved in how they're recorded. Makes my blood boil."

"Huh. I haven't thought much about it. My mom's keeping her own notes, in her own book. She writes down everything."

"Good." She unwrapped a syringe, looked at it carefully. "I'm going to give you a sedative before I start, OK? Stronger than the one you had earlier. Go ahead and give yourself a bump of the pain meds now, you won't be able to do it yourself once I get started."

He reached and pushed the button, as familiar to him now as his own thumb. "Done."

"Can you roll over onto your right side? Is that easier than your left?"

"Probably." He struggled to turn, twisting his upper half. Even with the meds, a shot of pain raced up his spine. "Oh my God. Any way you can do it with me on my back?"

Delilah looked over her glasses at him, then put down the syringe. "Let me get some help. Be right back."

When she returned, Ramón and another man came with her, looking unhappy to have been summoned. "He can't just hold it there on his own?" Ramón asked irritably.

"You'll have to do it for him. Hold him carefully. It's not a very comfortable position."

"God forbid he should be uncomfortable for a few minutes," Ramón shot back. Delilah gave him a look, which seemed to silence him for the time being. They turned him slowly, then, onto his side, the two men steadying him between them as they reached from alternate sides of the bed. Delilah pushed the syringe into one of the IV ports, held it there for a few seconds, then pulled it out and threw it away.

Almost instantly he felt transported to another place: an urban aqueduct of some sort, set deep below the streets above. He was horizontal to the water, just at its peak, holding onto the stone sides by his fingers and toes. The water rushed past, murky and warm, tugging at his hospital gown. He tried to reach back to hold it down but almost slipped and fell. He gripped harder, craning his neck to try to see over the top. Delilah appeared on the opposite side, just her shoulders and head. "Hold still, Patrick, hold still. I'm going in."

Suddenly some force tugged him forward, as if he was being pulled along a mechanical track. He could almost make it out just below the water's edge: big teeth and eyes, like an unwound cog, running along the wall. He seemed to be attached to it somehow, but he couldn't tell where. It tugged him forward again, moving in fits and starts.

"Almost done, but I need you to hold still," Delilah said, "just another minute. Right there. Don't move, OK?"

He tried to speak, tried to say, "Why are they doing this to me? Why here?" He wasn't sure if he had actually made the words or not; Delilah only said, "Almost done, almost done. There we go. Needle's out. *Gently*, guys, OK? Lay him *gently*."

In a flash he had fallen into the city river, felt it washing over him as he watched the sky: gray, too gray, like granite in a cave. He thought he saw people moving far above, near the edge of the stone wall, walking along as if none of this was happening. They seemed not to know he was there. He began yelling for them, trying to catch their attention, get some help to get him out.

"Patrick, *Patrick*." It was Delilah again, there she was craning over the wall, looking down at him, reaching for him. "Patrick, calm down. You're fine. We're done. Hold my hand."

He wasn't allowed dinner that night, in advance of the surgery. They'd brought him a late lunch, late as they could, then taken it away, quick as it came. He grew to dread those three letters posted above his bed: NPO. They haunted him, and even much later, long gone from that place, he would sometimes awake, dead of night, and scramble to look over the headboard, terrified that they had returned and were stopped there, waiting for him.

31

Morning came quick, and before he even felt fully awake they were rolling him away, down the hall and into a brightly lit room. Deirdre had walked with him, as far as she could. "Your father's flying in today," she said in those last moments. "Should be here by the time you're back in your room." He smiled at her through the haze, told her he loved her. And then she was gone, closed behind two doors that swung shut.

A profundity of movement, of silent preparation. Blue eyes above a blue mask, talking to him. "Mizrahi," he thought he heard the mask say, "almost ready. Start from one-hundred. Backwards, now ..." He got as far as ninety-eight. Whatever happened next was lost to him, stripped away forever by the amnesia-inducing drugs that they gave.

But then he was back, a different room now: white, with flecks of red and gray; drapes hung to the side; low, tonal beeps and whirs; and a head there, looking down at him, saying his name. "Wake up, there you go, there you go." He felt a rough pull in his throat, but then it was gone. "Good job, there you go." She was still looking down, smiling at him. "... recovery room, you're just waking up. Feel OK?"

"Nausea," he said.

She turned, rustling, and he heard a faint pop. He started to feel more stable, back on semi-solid ground. Things stopped their waving and stilled. Slowly, he caught on to time, like grabbing a rope, felt it moving and taking him with it.

"Good job," she said again. "Want a little water?" He nodded, and she produced a straw, put it between his lips, which felt dry and chaffed. "Just a little bit. One little sip." She withdrew the straw. "That's good, that's enough."

His mother appeared at the edge of his vision. "How are you feeling?" she asked. "Pain?"

He tried to speak, or thought he did, but she looked at him harder, repeated herself. "Yeah," he finally said, or heard himself say.

"Yeah you're in pain?"

"Yeah." Deirdre turned and said something he couldn't hear; more rustling and pops, and then a sweet wave washed over him, rinsing him out. He felt exceptionally clean and comfortably cool. He felt pristine, actually, brand new, just out of the box. He smiled widely and smoothly, a single long gesture, and allowed his eyes to drift shut.

Thirteen beds to a nurse meant that attentions were more lax here: less regular, less predictable, less sure. What's worse, this was the psych ward. Nurses acted differently, didn't trust the patients. When people's mental states are called into question, given names as disorders, conviviality falls away. It all moved by force; no options, no questions, just a sturdy forward-motion that factored out the question of agency, of deliberation, of being someone who might want to *decide*.

It wasn't the nurses' fault, not exactly; they too were told what to do. But the blanket feel of this place, its fragile sociality, was defined by containment rather than choice. Each one who worked with him, who visited him to take his vitals, draw his blood, check his fluids, softened just enough to acknowledge that he was being housed on the wrong floor. But still he could feel their resentment, could taste and smell it, could hear it in the way they moved up and down the ward. They were as miserable, as unfulfilled, as everyone else here.

He had slept through the night, knocked out by more tranquilizers and pain meds, dreamless in his dead weight. He had prepared himself for the difficult string of days, and imagined that this one, the day after the first incision had been made, would be the worst. If that was the case, maybe things wouldn't be so bad. He could feel, with sharp intensity, how serious the surgery had been: the wound was long, held temporarily closed by staples, wrapped in gauze that bore a faint line of red, a palimpsest of where they'd gone in. He could feel where they'd drilled, the dull roar of it where holes must now be. He sensed a compact pressure in his bone where they must have packed the beads—couldn't feel them exactly, but could tell something was there that hadn't been before.

Jonathan had arrived during the surgery. He was sitting here now; he had asked Deirdre if she would give them some time alone, and she had gone for a walk. "Patrick, I've asked some people to come visit you. They should be here any minute."

"You've what? Dad, I'm not really in a good place for visitors. Mom has a schedule, can you check with her?"

"This is a special group. From a church, down in Daly City. I contacted them from home. They want to come pray over you."

"Dad. I'm really not in a good place for visitors. I don't feel like seeing people."

"I thought it would be good for you, have local folks praying. They said they'd come visit you as often as you want, pray over you."

"I have a huge group of friends, Dad, people I already know, wanting to come visit. I don't have the energy for strangers."

Jonathan looked at his lap, disappointed in his son. Disappointed in himself. "What if they pray in the hall? Just outside?"

Patrick looked at his father. "I guess that would be fine. I'm sorry, Dad. I know you're trying to do what you can to help. I really do. And I appreciate it. I just don't feel like seeing people."

"That's OK, son, I understand." Jonathan was renewed by his idea, starting to imagine how he might frame this: he's very ill, the surgery was long, let's let him rest while we gather right outside his room. "I understand, I do." Deirdre walked into the room, smiled at them both. Jonathan stood up, shuffled over to the door, said: "I'm just gonna run downstairs, see if they're here yet."

"See if who's here yet?" Deirdre said, suddenly alarmed. "Jonathan?" But he was already on his way, moving quickly down the hall. She turned back to the room. "What's he talking about?"

"Apparently he called a local church. Asked some people to come pray over me. People I don't know."

"Are you kidding me?"

"No. I told him they couldn't come in, mom. He's just trying to help. Please, don't say anything."

She turned and looked out the door again, wondering if she could catch up with him, then turned back. "I can't believe him."

"Mom, really, he's just trying to help. Let him do what he can."

She closed her eyes, breathed in and let it back out. "I know. I know he is." She walked over to the window. "Did you remind him I have a schedule?"

"I did. I don't think he knew."

"Oh, he knew," she said. "He knew."

A few minutes later, there was a soft rustling at the door as Jonathan hurried in. "Patrick, they're here. Really nice guys, I mean it. You sure you don't feel like visitors?"

"I'm sure."

"OK, son, that's fine. We understand." He turned and looked down the hall, then back in the room. "I'll just close this door, OK? We'll meet out here for a few minutes. I'll be back." He walked out, pulling the door behind him. Patrick heard faint voices there, talking, and Jonathan's wide laughter filling the hall. Deirdre rolled her eyes. The door cracked open, and the nurse came in. He heard someone say "blood of Jesus" faintly, as if through an echo.

"What is *that*?" the nurse asked.

"That's my dad. He brought some people to pray for me. I just don't feel like seeing visitors, so they're doing it out there."

The nurse's face softened. "What a nice man," she said. "You take everything you can get, you hear? Take everything you can get. A little prayer from strangers never hurt anybody."

Patrick reached and pressed the button. "I know," he said, "I know."

He ate greedily at five, just before the cut-off. Meatloaf and mashed potatoes, surprisingly good. Deirdre and Jonathan sat in chairs four feet apart, watching him eat.

"Not too bad, really," he said. "I can definitely feel it, but if this is the worst, I'll be fine."

Deirdre was worried. Doctor Mizrahi had said the first day would be difficult, but that the following surgeries would happen in such quick succession that they might be worse. He wasn't sure. The only salvation was that it was a compact schedule, done in a week or ten days. She didn't think most of this had registered with Patrick. He seemed to have made up his mind that the first cut was the worst.

She imagined what would happen: that wound, the one made yesterday, would have just started to heal, bonding itself back together, when they'd pull it open again. And again, and again. It sounded horrific, like slow torture. She was worried that Patrick would face a steep and sharp decline, a complete dampening.

Jonathan was humming some tune or other, in good spirits. She had talked to him after the church group left, told him how important the schedule was; they both must stick to it. No exceptions. He'd listened carefully, cowed by having forgotten. But he'd rebounded quickly—really, she hadn't been rude at all, had actually been quite kind—telling her how nice the people were, how thoughtful to have come. "They don't know us from Adam," he said. "And ten people showed up. Salt of the earth. I tell you, Deirdre, salt of the earth."

Deirdre sent him back to his hotel that night, strict instructions to return by seven in the morning. He should be here when they were prepping Patrick for surgery, be here to walk with him down to the OR. "I'll be here," he said, "earlier if possible. Not sleeping well lately, not at all. My back's been acting up."

"Have you seen a doctor?" she asked.

"Oh yeah, seen a few. Runs in the family, you know, back trouble."

"Sorry to hear that," Deirdre said.

"I don't want the surgery," he said.

"No."

They looked together at their oldest son, who was writing on some paper his mother had given him, unaware of them watching. He was trying to describe what the wound felt like, the itch and throb of it. He was trying to narrate the recovery room, waking up. He was trying to give a feel for what this room was like, and the window, and the view outside. Before he went to sleep, he was trying to characterize, to give meaning to, this day-between, this suture, this middle-man in the process. He wasn't having much luck—the words wouldn't come—but he was trying anyway, refusing to give up.

32

It was a tumult, the day and what came after—a complete upheaval, again, in the flow that had slowly started to even itself out, get regular and remembered. Pre-op had been fine; mild sedative, then the trip downstairs, his parents following alongside. The goodbye again as the drip picked up its pace; the doctor's voice, the moving around, and once more the counting. This time he made it down to ninety-six.

But in the recovery room, as he was slowly dragged up and out of the fog, everything was different. His skin seemed to melt with every upward surge, softening then dripping around him, pooling on the bed. This sensation was followed by what can only be described as a tenderness, as with a bruise, enveloping his entire being, inside and out. Each cell threatened to burst if brushed against, every string and fiber awake and alert. A movement next to his bed, forcing the slightest breath of wind, scorched him, leaving a burn. His mouth was cranked open, head tilted back, as he attempted to cry out; but no sound came, not a whisper or shout.

The nurse upped his meds, watching him helplessly. She rang for the doctor, who thankfully had not yet left the floor. When he arrived, he hovered over Patrick's bed cautiously, watching him seize. "Do you think we should put him back under?" the nurse asked.

"I don't, no. He needs to wake up. We can help if he wakes up."

"I think he *is* awake," she said, "just unable to speak. He seems to be in a lot of pain."

This time that Patrick awoke, he overheard this conversation but could not participate in it. Every piece of him was on fire; but the worst of it was in his leg. Was someone slicing him open now? Had they forgotten to close the wound? He felt splayed, literally splayed, like a fish on the grill, laid open for all to see.

Gradually this feeling began to fade; the nurse was fidgeting with something near the IV, and Doctor Mizrahi was speaking to him. After a time, he could speak back. "It hurts, it hurts, it hurts, it hurts. Can you make it stop, it hurts so much, please …" And then it started to fall away, taking him with it. He sank back further into the bed as his skin seemed slowly to re-congeal, pulling itself back into its proper shape, back into its proper place. It wrapped itself around him, filling his nooks and crannies, softening the sting everywhere. And now he was groggy, overcome with grogginess, like a hangover, like the flu, like a profoundly disturbing dream.

"Better?" Doctor Mizrahi asked, looking down at him, knowing somehow not to touch him.

"Less bad," Patrick said, coming back to himself.

Being pushed through the halls like nothing had happened, he caught quick glimpses of those pock-marked tiles on the ceiling before trying to close it all out. He thought he saw Delilah walking past, thought he caught her wink, but this might just have been a memory. Nothing seemed the same; the very building was inverted somehow, as if he were in the mirror-image of it rather than in the place itself. *Everything* seemed inverted, folded inside-out, the opposite of what it should be. Mostly he felt wet, like his insides were unnaturally drenched. He wondered if he was feeling his own blood, or maybe the water of his cells. He wondered if he was bleeding, if that's what this was.

There was a tube sticking out of the wound, a drain. After the first surgery, he had gotten used to it there, doing its slow work. It meant he could move even less than before; but he didn't mind. Now it seemed like a vacuum, pulling the very life out of him, sucking it dry. More than anything he wanted to yank it out, but he was not so delirious as to try this. He knew he couldn't. And somehow his insides itched, as if the underside of his skin had had some reaction, poison ivy or oak. He imagined himself rubbing calamine lotion there, on the inside surface of his skin. He wondered: is it a surface? Would that even make sense? Or is it all of a piece, shoved up so close to everything else that it isn't practically distinguishable? He drifted off again, feeling himself roll through the halls, the bumps when they crossed a threshold to another ward, the shift in buoyancy when they entered the lift and rode to the next floor, and the next, and the next after that.

And it only got worse. That night he barely spoke, barely slept. The day between was a blur of agony and angst. He could not register what Doctor Mizrahi was saying during his visits; could not carry a conversation with Deirdre or Jonathan; was not aware of the revolving-door of nurses coming and going, in and out like shoppers in a corner market. He barely spoke at all, except to say "yes" and "no" when prompted. He had no sense of time, or of place, or of where he was in the world. The pain was technically managed; but his discomfort was absolute. He would shift constantly for long periods, trying to find a position that would not offend, and then lie still for a while, until the pressure points became too much to handle—and so he would shift again, no relief to be found, no repose to intervene. The third surgery was completely transparent in its full-throated attack.

Unlike the first time he awoke, and the period that followed, this was not a fantastical series of days: he rarely dreamed, unable to sleep for more than an hour at a time. And he did not experience visits, or the figure of Deirdre sitting constantly by his side, as anything more than mere fact. Nothing embroidered his days or nights; it was a coldly clinical time, like a crime scene at dawn. Things simply happened, and happened differently, and happened again. No escape, no excuse, nothing to dull the profoundly intolerable boredom of the ride.

He gave himself over to it finally, existing in compliance with the expectation that things must go on and we might as well let them. On the day before the fourth of these surgeries, Doctor Mizrahi came to visit at four in the afternoon. "Patrick," he said, "this is it."

"This is *what?*"

"This is the last one. The last of these surgeries." He had sent Deirdre and Jonathan away, and was sitting now like he did on that first day here, holding Patrick's hand and looking down at him solicitously.

Patrick lifted himself—felt himself lifting himself—just enough to indicate closer involvement in the conversation. "And do you think they're working? Is the infection going away? Is everything doing what you'd hoped?"

"I'm sorry to say this, but no. It's not." Doctor Mizrahi tilted his head slightly, almost maternal in the composure of his concern. "We haven't been able to make much progress."

Patrick sank back into the bed, grateful for the doctor's candor, but resigned now to sharp disappointment and a new prognosis that seemed suddenly to shimmer, twist, and collapse on top of him. "Oh."

"The infection is just too extensive. These bacteria ... they're relentless. They're not immune to the beads, but as a whole they are not responsive in the way we would hope."

"Oh."

"And the integrity of the bone—well, it's just not there. The bone is extraordinarily fragile. Profoundly fragile. Like brittle wood, threatening to splinter with every move."

"Oh. OK."

"So tomorrow's surgery is going to be a comma, not a period."

Patrick looked up at him sharply. "What?"

"I said, tomorrow will be a comma, not a period. We're going to have to try something else. Tomorrow I will go in and remove the beads that are there, but unless I see that things have changed dramatically, I won't put any more in."

"What *will* you do?"

"Send you down the road. To another hospital—your third, now, right? Or fourth? Anyway, you'll see another surgeon, a colleague of mine."

"What will *he* do?"

"I'll let him talk to you about what he thinks is best. But he will need to remove some of the bone. It will be necessary for him to do so. That much I can tell you."

"When will all of this happen?"

"The last surgery here will be tomorrow morning, early. Just like the others. It will be faster than those, though, and—again, unless things have changed by the time I go in—will be over quickly. Tomorrow night we'll move you to over to the next hospital. And the surgery with Doctor Blatt will be the following morning."

"So another surgery, only one day later?"

"That's right."

Patrick's eyes lost focus, making the world an impressionist's watercolor, a blur. "OK."

Doctor Mizrahi squeezed his hand. "Listen. Doctor Blatt can be off-putting. I've heard he can seem quite pessimistic when talking with patients. But he is a *very* talented surgeon, skilled with exactly this kind of work. I cannot think of anyone in the country who is similarly experienced, *no one* who is as successful as he is in resolving extremely complex cases. Keep this in mind, OK?"

"I'll try." He paused. "I'm feeling pretty fragile myself. Like I might splinter, too."

Doctor Mizrahi squeezed his hand again. "I know, Patrick. I know. I will be thinking of you, checking up on you through Blatt." He squeezed his hand again, then leaned over and kissed Patrick on the forehead. It was entirely unexpected, this move, and left Patrick feeling suddenly quite warm—but simultaneously completely broken, in constant need of continuous care. The doctor stood and turned to leave, letting Deirdre back into the room as he went out into the hall. As she rushed to enter, moving apace to the bed, Patrick became aware that his cheeks and face were drenched with tears he hadn't even known were there. They rolled and rolled out of him as if he held a bottomless reservoir of them, as if there were no end to their reproduction, as if they would not ever cease to flow.

Interlude

We were hungry again. In the periods between these rapid-fire interventions, left briefly to our own devices, we sped up our pace, devouring these moments of freedom as if they were a final meal. And though those beads were no doubt deadly, they were also familiar to us: we knew their method from family legends, passed through our very cells.

That story you've heard, about forgotten bread and a moldy spore, isn't exactly true. We'll tell it as it's been handed down, one generation to the next, among those strands of our family tree that have learned and taught us how to survive it. The famed Scotsman had a plate of our ancestors in his basement lab, which he had absent-mindedly left uncovered. One morning he saw, there in the dish, a small spot of mold; and around it, those of our family who had been nearest began to die—a circle of slaughter, extending out from the spot—and those too far beyond its reach to feel its effects were thriving from less competition. There were two lessons in this discovery: the first, of course, is that we have our sensitivities, our poisons, too; but the second, often forgotten, is that we learn how to endure, so that what was first poison becomes not merely harmless, but a kind of leverage. What was once toxic can give us an edge.

It took two years for anyone to be able to use this mold practically, as a cure. And even then the samples were too small, too impure, to have broad effect on more than a handful of the ill. Producing it in volumes sufficient for treatment, especially for large numbers of people, proved an insurmountable feat for ten years and more. By then you were immersed in your own flagrant war, spread across continents; and when the countless battle wounds from your own artillery shells, your own ammunitions, became hosts to our kin, you expanded your search for modes to manufacture the stuff on such a large scale that it could cover the globe. Unsatisfied with a war of the plainly visible world, you declared war on us.

The breakthrough was made by a woman in Illinois, a lab worker obsessed with the task, who sought and bought old produce from markets in town, soft and molding, bringing them back for tireless testing. She discovered one such golden growth on a melon, in a ring near its end, which turned out to be the key. Of course, she is not remembered as central to this story. You eulogized her as Moldy Mary, when you deigned to mention her at all.

And then you mass-produced the potion, used it promiscuously, spreading it out like a final cure. You assumed that we were too basic—too dumb—to respond with anything other than resignation. But we are a diverse and complex family; and many of us are able, at will, to defuse the effects of that drug, just by releasing a tiny signal—a trick to confuse and disarm. You reacted with shock—with immodest disbelief. You began to learn our language, a chemical grammar that keeps us working as a team. You began trying to use it against us, like deeply embedded spies who have trained in the details of dialect.

And we, in turn, learned your dialects, too; and each time they changed, we gave ourselves over to acculturation. Like anthropologists deep in the field, with every new deviation we grew slowly but doggedly to feel at home.

PART V

33

The fourth surgery was finished by ten o'clock, not that Patrick would have known. He was coaxed up and out of catatonia for the last time in this recovery room by the same nurse who had awakened him after each of the other operations. She was somber and still, standing by his bed with her right hand on his arm—always his arm—rubbing a small stretch of skin with her thumb. "You're in the recovery room, Patrick," she told him again. "You're just waking up. Can you open your eyes?"

They fluttered to life, looking up and around, as he slowly came to. He did not fight the awakening, did not react to its occurrence with anything more than a small nod. His eyes came to rest on a point behind her head: a ceiling tile, from his point of view, dotted with those tiny holes, arranged in a neat and orderly grid.

"I've given you an anti-emetic, just in case," she said. "Do you feel alright?"

He nodded again, a blatant lie—which she knew. She reached and gave him a small dose of the pain meds with her left hand, the right thumb still rubbing in place. His eyes glazed further.

"Can you tell me where you are?"

"Recovery room," he said slowly, wide spaces between the syllables and words. He sounded it out again, articulating each letter distinctly: "re-co-ver-y roo-m."

"Right. Good. Your surgery went well. Didn't take long. Your mom is waiting in the hall. Can I bring her in now? Do you want to see her?" He nodded slowly, pronouncing each movement of his head as a separate act.

The day passed slowly, winding its way through his room with tender if tardy efficiency. He stared at the walls, at the ceiling, occasionally at the floor. He allowed himself to close his eyes for twenty minutes at a time, pretending to sleep. It seemed not to matter if he was conscious or not; the slow crawl of minutes and hours continued at the same plodding pace, inching forward and around him, taking their time. The room filled with sunlight, then grayed over, then darkened completely. Those letters were there, marking terrain: NPO. He could feel them behind him, could sense their gentle pulse, like neon in an all-night café. He was fed through a tube, nutrients and protein, devised just to sustain.

When night had fully dropped, the bleached light of the overheads covering him and the room, paramedics arrived—not two but three this time, one in training. Doctor Mizrahi met them at the door. "Paperwork's here, in duplicate. He needs to go quickly: they're holding a bed, but they won't hold it forever." He walked back to Patrick, leaned down. "Good luck. I'll keep in touch. I'll be thinking of you. Stay with us, OK?" Patrick nodded.

Deirdre, huddled in the hall with the bags, stood watching the scene. Jonathan had left earlier in the day, rushed to get back to some pressing emergency at his church: an ill elder, readied for the grave. Deirdre motioned to the paramedics that she would be on her way so as to meet them there. She walked briskly but downcast, watching the floor. Her mouth was shut firmly, but her eyes were sharp and fixed. Her breaths came in short bursts, as if in formation for a processual. Remarkably, people seemed to move out of her way, acknowledging her path, sending her off with dignified bows. She rode the elevator alone, and marched through the parking garage in utter solitude, as if it had been cleared intentionally, as if it were a private space.

The new hospital was bright, decorous, and clean. In contrast to the cramped halls and rooms of General, this place was immaculate. It actually resembled a recently constructed resort: high ceilings with warm, recessed lighting; wide, respectable wards like wings of an estate; large windows overlooking a lush and open urban park. He marveled at the relative speed with which he was removed from the ambulance and wheeled directly to a room; only one brief stop at a broad, clean welcome desk, then a straight shot to a space that felt, in comparison, like a suite. Deirdre was already there. She had turned a window seat into a makeshift altar, decorating it with cards, flowers, pictures, the tree. He saw two new balloons drifting lazily around the window. Where did they come from? Why were they here? "Get Well Soon!" they both said, one with a series of ever-growing hearts in pink and red, the other with a dippy cartoon dog holding a thermometer in its mouth and an icepack to its head. He smiled in spite of himself, in spite of it all: she must have made a special stop to buy them.

The nurses here seemed more professional somehow, like First Class stewards on a transpacific flight. Two of them walked in now, greeting the paramedics with handshakes and smiles. "Welcome," they said. "We'll take those papers. Thank you." The paramedics, unfazed by the stark differences in decorum, gave signatures quickly and shuffled off. One of the nurses followed behind them, while the other began looking through Patrick's chart.

"Patrick, I'm Felicia. I'll be your nurse tonight. I've already met your mother. How are you feeling?" Patrick glanced up to see a tall, sturdy woman with long black dreadlocks, done up in a loose bun. She wore sharp cat-eye glasses, secured by an iridescent chain around her neck.

"I feel slow, weighed down. And hungry."

"I'm sure you do! Unfortunately I can't bring you any food. But I'll get your IV hooked up now. Doctor Blatt approved giving you a nutritional shake, which I'll send down for now. Favorite flavor?"

"Strawberry? Or peanut butter. Or whatever, I don't care."

"We've got strawberry."

"OK."

Felicia went to the phone, pressed a button, and placed the order. "Like room service," he thought. "How strange."

"How's your pain?"

"Endless."

"Any different from when you left General?"

He thought about this for a moment, focusing on each constitutive part of his body briefly before answering. "Not really."

"How would you describe it?"

"Dull. Throbbing. Deep."

"OK. I'm going to go ahead and start your pain meds. You know how to use this, right?" She held up the wand, gesturing to the button.

"Yeah."

"Good. Stay ahead of it, OK?"

"Yeah."

She was fast and methodical with the IV needle, had it in and taped up before he was even aware of her fiddling with his arm. She turned to the pain machine, checked its settings, then closed and locked its little transparent door. "OK, it should be set. Go ahead and give it a try."

He pressed the button gingerly, not out of concern for its sensitivity, but because he could not quite muster the enthusiasm to be more direct. Within seconds he could feel that now-familiar swell of relief.

"Oh—oh, yes, it's working. I can feel it. Thank you." Being without the medication, even for the relatively short time it took the paramedics to load him up, transport him, and drop him off again in this place—just over two hours—meant that he had grown accustomed to the growing thrum of the systemic ache; this made the relief all that much more extensive.

"Good. I'll be back in a few minutes. We're five beds to a nurse, so I won't be long. Just call if you need me."

"OK."

A small man, wiry and quick, popped into the room: "Delivery from the kitchen? For Mister Anderson? Strawberry shake?"

"Yes. Leave it with him. Thanks, Don," Felicia said, and then she was gone, and then they both were gone. Deirdre twisted open the small bottle, fed a straw into it, and then handed it to Patrick.

"Drink slowly. Try to space it out. This is all you can have tonight."

The first sip transported him instantly to childhood: sitting on that brown speckled carpet, Saturday mornings, cartoons on the old television, strawberry milk in an adult-size glass. He remembered his brother, sitting next to him. He remembered a stuffed bear squeezed between his arms, held down by the glass as he drank from it. He remembered the feel of the milk on his lip, held as a dripping mustache against his skin. He remembered the sensation of licking it off, once the drink was gone, and holding on to those last few drops, the flavor staying with him through the long day until he was rewarded—sometimes, not every night—with a second glass before bed.

Doctor Blatt did not visit that night, but sent one of his residents, a tall man with glasses, a swimmer's build, and skin the distinct color of a very pale nectarine. He was wearing a suit, three piece, beneath his doctor's robe; he couldn't have been older than thirty.

"Did Doctor Mizrahi explain what we're going to do? Or your doctor ..." he looked at his notes, "Doctor Pettle?"

"Yes, a little bit. But can you explain it again?"

"I'll do better than that!" the man said, his enthusiasm set at an inappropriate level for the occasion. "I'll draw you a picture!" He pulled a yellow legal pad out of his bag, as if preparing for a high school debate competition. In bright blue ink, he began to sketch the shape of a femur: its narrowing, oddly cylindrical descent from hip to knee. At the top, set at about a forty-five degree angle from the central vertical line, he drew the little oval head, then surrounded that curve with a perfectly mirrored casing: the cup of the hip. "Here is your leg," he said, pointing with the pen to the femur. "And here is your hip." He moved the pen in quick circles around the joint, leaving a darkening halo around it. "Now let's blow this part up."

Patrick looked up at the man. "Excuse me?"

"Oh—ha-ha! I mean, let me draw a bigger version. Like on a map!"

He enlarged the image by re-sketching it to the side. Patrick watched his face as he did this, trying not to show his distrust.

"There we go! OK, so this part of the bone is infected, as you know." Patrick looked back down at the paper, where the doctor was drawing a series of cross-hatched designs inside the femoral head. "And there's a little infection maybe spreading between these bones, into the pelvis. All of the cartilage here is lost. Totally gone. That's why you've been in so much pain—the direct friction of bone-on-bone. Well, that and the fact that the bacteria are eating away the inside of your femur." He re-drew a new set of cross-hatches on top of the originals, extending them down the bone.

"Got it," Patrick said.

"So tomorrow we're going to go in and cut this all out." He drew a sharp line across the bone, separating the femoral head and about a quarter of the main shaft. "Ordinarily we wouldn't take so much; but we want to cut well below the infection line, just to make sure we get it all."

This exercise was beginning to seem to Patrick like a battlefront tête-à-tête drawn out on a parchment map: a battalion of invaders, lines of attack, plans for defense. "Yes, sir," he said militaristically. The doctor didn't get it, or didn't care to respond.

"We'll also need to debride some muscle around here—whatever's infected or dead. And then we'll put in a temporary prosthesis, which—this is really cool, actually—we make right in the operating room, using your old bone as a model! It'll be made of a special kind of cement, imbedded and coated with antibiotics. It won't be weight-bearing, so you can't really walk on it."

"I understand."

"That'll stay in for a while—probably six weeks or so. Then we'll go in and do it again, maybe even a third time. Just to make sure the infection's treated."

"Got it."

"And finally, we'll replace the cement with metal—which *will* be weight-bearing."

"OK. Got it."

"Any questions about any of this?"

"Am I in the hospital that whole time?"

"Oh no. No, no, no. You'll go home a few days, maybe a week, after this surgery. Then you'll come back for the replacement, go home again, and so on, and then back for the final procedure—what we *hope* will be the final procedure."

"OK."

"And that's it! You'll be good as new."

"Good as new."

"Sure you don't have any questions?"

"I don't think so. Mom?"

"I'm good." Deirdre was writing this all down. "Can I keep that drawing?"

"Of course you can! Wait, let me sign it, ha-ha!" He scribbled his name, which Patrick hadn't caught, and tore the page off his pad. "Here you go."

"When do I meet Doctor Blatt?"

"He'll see you in pre-op. He does a *lot* of surgeries—just got out of one now—so he can't see you before that."

"OK. Thanks."

"Alright! See you in the morning, Patrick. Well—you won't see me, but I'll be seeing you! Keep up that bravery, OK?" The doctor smiled and walked out of the room, a bounce in his step.

Patrick looked at Deirdre, who quickly rolled her eyes. "Good Lord," she said.

He smiled. "What the hell *was* that?" And for the first time in so long they couldn't remember, they lost themselves in laughter, knowing full well this might be their last chance for a while. Deirdre actually doubled over, clutching her legs. She infused herself with laughter when it came like this, skin flushed and pulsing, eyes like a monsoon, mouth stretched so wide she felt it might rip apart at the seams, baring her teeth. They laughed wildly, maniacally, hysterically, and did not want it ever to fade away.

34

"I understand everything has been explained to you," said Doctor Blatt. He was wearing surgical scrubs, a protective hat, and gloves on his hands. He balanced one arm on the rail of the gurney and leaned into it, casually crossing one leg over the other as if standing at a bar.

"Yes, last night."

"Good. This is Maria, my assistant. She'll be in the OR with me, and she'll be the one checking on you most often once it's done."

Maria stood to the side of the doctor in identical scrubs. Her eyes were fixed on him, seeming to hold him in their attention, and she smiled comfortably; Patrick thought he picked up the slightest sense of apology from her, knowing full well how abrasive the doctor could be.

"Hi, Maria," he said.

Before she could respond, Doctor Blatt reached over him and grabbed the file, balanced precariously on the table next to him. "Let me just check something quickly." He flipped through a few pages. "Good. You didn't eat yesterday."

"Just the shake."

"Right. OK, off we go. Deirdre? Deirdre—this will take about six hours, maybe longer. He'll be in recovery sometime this afternoon, back in his room by early evening."

"Will he be able to have dinner?" Deirdre asked. She was not impressed by the doctor's tone, but she hid her disfavor like a professional.

"Sure. No problem. As long as he gets out of recovery on time."

"But I could bring him something from outside, if he's too late for the kitchen here?"

"Yeah, that's fine. I'll let you know if I change my mind. Maria, let's go."

He turned and began hustling away; Maria reached down, squeezed Patrick's shoulder: "We'll take good care of you, OK?" And then she turned to follow the doctor out of the room.

"You OK?" Deirdre asked.

"Yeah. What a jerk."

"I know. Let's just hold on to what everyone has said: that he's very good at this. Maria seems nice. Hopefully she'll be there whenever you talk to him."

"I hope so. What a jerk."

The nurse pushed lorazepam into the IV, soothing him into a tranquil sea at low tide. "Almost ready for you, Patrick." She unlocked the wheels of the bed, pulled him out slightly from the wall, moved the curtain, and pushed him further into the room. He was surrounded by little areas, draped off into cubicles, with people lying on beds like his, family members standing nearby. A lot of waiting, plenty of worry. Someone was crying softly on the other side, to his right. He could hear her sniffs and sighs, tapering off as he was wheeled away, as if drifting back into the depths of a sound-proof room.

They went through double doors that had swung open as they'd approached. A large, sterile anteroom greeted them there, with spigots and sinks occupying small areas along the way. He could see a second set of double doors coming, saw them begin to open as they grew close, then became overwhelmed with the bright gleam of light on the other side: like sliding into the center of light itself, this travel. Like riding a beam all the way back to its source.

This time he dreamed—not during the surgery itself, but as he was starting to wake. He was on a great slide, moving quickly down, watching the scenery below from an intense height. The air was cool and damp, as if he were moving through clouds; but the view was clear and unobstructed by haze or fog. He could see patches of green skirting the edge of a lake, rising and falling as the ground swelled with hills and canyons. No one was there; it was deserted, or untouched. He neither sped nor slowed as he moved, just keep the same pace despite the length of the fall. It was enormously pleasant, even fun, as he went down. And it seemed never to end: he could not see a terminus, could not sense where he would finally land. And there was no anxiety in this, no worry about what was happening.

He was smiling openly, his mouth in the shape of a large bowl, as he awoke. He wasn't laughing, exactly, but made a long, joyful sound, like "Aaaah ..." that ebbed and flowed as he withdrew slowly from the dream and returned back into the world. "Aaaah..." he breathed again as his eyelids rose to the foggy view of a woman watching him wake.

"Look who's back!" she said cheerfully, reading the signs.

"Aah ... uh. Woah," he replied. He looked quickly around the room, turning his head.

"Careful, now. Careful," she said. "Thirsty?"

They went through the motions, taking each step of waking as he had taken them before: the small sips of water, the slow sitting up, bringing in Deirdre, then finally getting packed in and being moved away. He was struck by the ritual of it, by its dependable happening over and over, just as it always did, in exactly the same order.

"This isn't nearly as fun," he said as his bed was pushed through the halls, "as that slide."

The orderly, an older man with frosty white hair, wasn't bothered. "Want me to go faster?"

"Nah, thanks, it still won't be the same."

Deirdre trailed along behind them. She had spoken briefly with Doctor Blatt in the recovery room while Maria checked on Patrick. She was trying to get everything he'd said down in her book, but she couldn't remember all of the technical terms, the jargon, and was having to improvise. "Removed one-third of the bone. Infection everywhere, bone brittle. Removed large sections of muscle, gray and dead. Scraped away inside surface of hip, clearing it out.

Cement prosthetic, not weight-bearing. Will not walk." This last part almost stopped her cold: Doctor Blatt had told her that Patrick would not walk again. "Start shopping for wheelchair."

They arrived at the room, still stunning in size, and the orderly followed protocol: position the bed, lock the wheels, plug it all in. Deirdre couldn't get those words out of her head: "Won't walk again." They echoed, the doctor's voice seeming to bounce from all quarters of her brain. "Won't walk again, won't walk again," they taunted, leading her on.

It was early evening. Felicia was back on shift, assigned to Patrick for another night. She came into the room almost immediately after the orderly left: they were so punctual here, so meticulous and organized. "How's the patient?" she said. "Hungry?"

"Oh my God I am so hungry. Am I allowed to eat again?"

"Doctor says yes, so let's get you fed. Kitchen's closing before too long—so make your choices fast, OK?" She handed Patrick a menu—a *menu!*—with space for him to check off his selections.

He held the paper up very close to his eyes, only inches away: "Can I have all of it?" he asked.

"Nope. One salad, one entree, one side, one dessert."

"Can't you pretend there are two of us in this room? Just for tonight?" He grinned up at her.

"Wish I could."

"Alright, OK, let's do mixed greens, spaghetti—extra cheese, please—and green beans. Cheesecake for dessert."

When the meal arrived—less than twenty minutes—he ate as he had never eaten before: in one fell swoop. The food was gone, plate licked clean, within ten minutes.

"I tried to tell him to slow down," Deirdre told Felicia.

"That's OK. As long as he's not nauseated, he'll be fine. I get it—he's hungry."

Doctor Blatt walked through the door, no knock or introduction, with Maria close behind. "Well, listen guys, it was very bad—even worse than we thought."

Felicia turned and looked at him, then quietly loaded the dirty dishes and flatware on the tray to take it away.

"Was it?" Patrick asked sheepishly.

"Very bad. The bone was dead—I don't know *why* Mizrahi even bothered trying to save it. And there was a lot of dead muscle. No saving any of it. But we got it all out, got rid of it."

There was a slight pause as Deirdre and Patrick passed a look.

"And you put in the cement thing?"

"Yes. I did a great job shaping it, and it fit perfectly. We'll be able to work out any length issues later. You know not to try to put too much weight on it, right?"

"That's what you said, yes."

"You can stand, but whenever you do you'll need to use a walker. Use your arms to hold the weight. You could do a lot of damage to yourself if you put too much on it."

"I understand."

"Better to get used to the wheelchair anyway."

"Why? What do you mean?"

"Well, I mean, you're going to be using one from here on out. So you might as well get accustomed to it."

"Using one what? A wheelchair?"

"Yeah. You're done with walking."

Patrick felt a sudden, sharp sense of vertigo. "Are you serious?"

Doctor Blatt took a step closer to the bed and seemed to puff out his chest. "I'm completely serious. I'm trying to save your *life* here, Patrick. You're lucky I didn't amputate the whole leg today. Keep that in mind."

Patrick just looked at him, willing himself not to respond. Doctor Blatt held his gaze, then turned away and looked down at his notes.

"Anyway. I'll check on you tomorrow. We'll want to get you up and out of here quickly. You'll come into my office for appointments every two weeks, then come back for another surgery in six. Deirdre, good night. Good night, Patrick."

He turned and left, leaving Maria behind. She walked quickly to Patrick and kneeled down next to the bed. "Listen. He's abrupt, and can be hard to stomach sometimes. You're going to be fine. We'll find you a good physical therapist. No telling what you'll be able to do." She smiled at Deirdre, then turned back to him. "If you're anything like your mom, I bet you'll be *running* before everything's said and done. Just focus on now, OK?"

"Thanks," Patrick said. His eyes were red again, bulging even as he willed them to stay tidy. "Thank you. Thank you so much."

"You bet," Maria said. "Now get a good night's sleep, and I'll see you tomorrow. She stood, reached over to squeeze his hand, and then turned to go.

"What a *jerk* that man is," Deirdre said.

Patrick reached for the button, pressed it again. He had already forgotten the doctor, put him out of his mind. "I can't believe how different I feel."

"How so?" Deirdre asked.

"Smoothed out. Like there's something gone from me, something that had been squeezing my insides, tugging at them, pulling me inward and down. It's hard to explain."

"And now?"

"Well, like it's just been unwound, whatever that was. Like it's been released."

"That seems good, right?"

"Oh, yes. I mean, I can still feel that things aren't quite right. And there's still pain—I can tell it's there, under the drugs. The drain, I don't know, it's a weird feeling, too. But the tightness is gone, the tension. Just gone."

Deirdre wrote these things down in her book, watching the words as she formed them on each page, as if they had a life of their own.

35

There was a small gathering of souls in his room, hours after he had awoken, taken breakfast, and been bathed and re-dressed in a fresh gown. The bedsheets had been replaced, too, and felt like crisp slices of cotton paper. He liked the feel of them, moved his right foot gently back-and-forth in appreciation of their flat, cool simplicity. Deirdre was here, and Doctor Pettle, and Tugboat Tim, and Robin, and Jan. They were perched on chairs dragged in from down the hall.

Felicia had gone off-shift, replaced by someone new: Marcus, he'd said when he first came in, and he didn't put up with any funny business. Patrick had looked at him skeptically—like "what in the world would I *do*?"—then watched as he broke a spacious smile. "Just kidding, Patrick. Just pulling your leg ... I mean ... uh." He'd briefly looked concerned, unsure how diligent Patrick was with feeling the seriousness of his state.

"Good thing," Patrick replied. "It might pop off." And then Marcus had laughed, a boisterous, unusually low-pitched laugh, like a bassoon gone haywire.

"I don't want all of this news spread to everyone, OK?" Patrick said to Robin. "I mean, you can tell people that I made it through the first surgery but, please, no specifics as to what they're doing."

"Sure thing, honey," Robin replied, taking notes. "Can I tell them you'll have to come back for more?"

"Oh yeah, of course. That's fine. Give a sense of the schedule. I just don't want details about the surgeries out there. People start writing or calling with questions and advice, stuff they heard or read somewhere. And—I don't know how to put this—I don't want the knowing looks all the time from everybody. The sympathetic head-tilts. Creeps me out."

"You bet. You want me to send it to you first? So you can approve it before it goes out?"

"No, no—I actually don't want to see it at all, not ever."

Robin looked at Jan, who then turned to Patrick. "No problem," she said. "I've been saving them all, printing them out and keeping them in a folder, just in case you ever change your mind. But we'll keep you off the list."

"Thanks."

Robin looked over at Deirdre. "Do we know when he's going to be released? People want to do things for him once he's back home. Bring food, spend the night if need be, stuff like that."

"Probably next week," she said. "The wound needs to heal enough, the drain needs to come out, and he needs to pass some physical therapy tests before they'll discharge him."

"Are you going to stay while he's home? Between the surgeries?"

Deirdre looked over at Patrick. "We haven't talked about it yet. I'll need to go home at some point, get some things done there, get back to the office. I don't know for how long, or when."

Patrick watched her, suddenly aware of how much time must have passed since she'd first arrived: three months? Four? Had she really been here all that time? He felt a sudden pang of embarrassed gratitude, like he'd asked too much—or hadn't *asked*, exactly, but needed without asking. Somehow that made it worse, made him feel even more cowed by her help.

Marcus returned to the room just then, clapped his hands and started rubbing them together. "OK, folks, we need to get him up. Can y'all clear out for a few minutes? I'm just gonna take him on a little walk. Not too long."

They all shuffled out of their chairs, began moving towards the door. Tim stopped at the bed, said: "Hey little prince, I've gotta get back to the marina. I'll give you a call later, OK? Try to stop by again tomorrow or the next day."

"OK. Thanks for coming."

"Glad to do it. Especially with you feeling a little better." He leaned down and left a small peck on Patrick's cheek, rubbed his hair with one bold, creased hand.

Once they were all gone, Marcus lowered the bars on the bed and began teaching Patrick how to move, a distinct choreography of shift, turn, shift, turn that reminded Patrick, fleetingly, of an old children's game. He had a brief flash of memory: moving, then holding in place when someone called "red light," trying to freeze.

The moving was not painful, but it was draining. Every inch seemed to take the wind out of him, as if he'd run a full mile. Once he'd reached the edge of the bed, and his legs were hanging down to the floor, Marcus reached around him in a giant bear hug: "OK, now, slowly, slowly, Patrick, bring yourself up. I've got the walker right next to me."

The indignity of this—being coached how to walk, using *that* device in particular—touched but did not settle on him. He shook it off willfully, insistently.

Once he was vertical, Marcus slowly released him, allowing him to stand on his own, his arms pressingly forcefully into the arms of the walker. "Your arms are quite strong, actually," Marcus said. "Probably because you've been using them so much. Do you feel stable?"

"Yeah," Patrick said, panting, "but winded."

"That's to be expected. OK, so, you can slide the walker ahead of you, then step—carefully, though. First step with your right leg, weight on it. Don't put too much on your left."

Patrick did as he was told, and made three slow steps before stopping again. "Uh," he said. "Tired."

"That's OK, take a rest before the next step. You're doing great. Keep it up. We're just gonna move over to the armchair, have you sit up for a while."

"Yeah," Patrick said, waiting, "OK." He took another step, then stopped and waited again.

"Good job, Patrick. Just a few more." Marcus moved to place a hand on the small of Patrick's back, not steadying him, but just letting him know that it was there.

Patrick progressed, one step at a time. His legs began to feel heavy, like they were pooling blood. They started to drag slightly, just as he made it round to the chair.

"Great, Patrick. Great. Now we're going to turn, just pivot in place—no, no, not your body. Pivot the walker. Think like a clock, you at the center. Turn the walker to three o'clock … good, that's right … now six o'clock. Good. Keep going, all the way around, until your back is facing the chair. Good, good. Now, bend slowly at the waist—slowly, Patrick, as slow as you can. Lean back into the chair. You're close enough, don't worry. It'll catch you. Not too fast."

This continued until Patrick was fully seated. Marcus reached around and pulled a lever, which tilted the chair back and raised a footrest from its base.

"That's it. Good job, Patrick. You made it. You made it." He pulled a small towel from somewhere and began wiping the sweat from Patrick's face. "Fantastic. Chair feel OK?"

"Yeah," Patrick said. He looked at his arm, where the IV was plugged, its tubes now stretched slightly across from the rack and machine. He was surprised to see how short a distance he had traveled—not even long enough to require that things be rolled closer to him. Right next to the bed, really. Just a few feet.

"This gonna get easier?" he asked, still out of breath.

"Bet on it."

Over the coming days, there would be an endless supply of small trainings: not just walking, such as it was, but smaller, discrete tasks, like picking things up, getting dressed, tying his shoes. Everything seemed to require a specific technique, one that wasn't intuitive or obvious. It all had to be learned, each with the help of an expert, a professional, a guide. And most moves required tools: a wide variety of hooks, claws, gripping devices, stiff loops. He was collecting a full supply of them, gathered neatly in a long bag set discreetly by the bed.

The trainings were terrifically boring; he had to focus on the smallest gestures, the slightest movements, of which there seemed to be so many more than one might think. Every crease and bend, the placement of hands, the arch and flex of feet, the shift at the waist, had to be demonstrated, mimicked, rehearsed over and over until they became a kind of second-nature, the body moving without thinking.

That was the goal, at least: training his body to work on its own. But for him, as he went through the performance of standing up, balancing to put on a shirt or leaning to pull on some socks, he remained conscious of each tiny flick of the wrist, of every single bend at the back. Like complex mathematics, like learning a new spoken tongue, he had to think through every gesture, imagine its occurrence as it was playing out. On one hand this gave him something to do; it took up time by occupying his mind. But on the other it was tedious, dampening, and sharply disquieting, especially when such careful practice culminated in success on such a small scale: the socks were on; the shoe was tied; he was seated now someplace else.

Doctor Pettle stuck around for Doctor Blatt's return; he wanted to meet the man and run interference. Deirdre had explained how short his temper seemed, how caustic and bitter his presence felt. It was, as it happens, a short visit, in and out in under five minutes. Maria was not with him this time, busy tending to someone else.

"It was a very good incision," Doctor Blatt said, inspecting the wound. "Not too much drainage. I have Mizrahi to thank for that, I suppose. Hard to believe, looking at it, but it's been used five times now to enter you."

"When will the staples come out?" Patrick asked, trying not to think about what the doctor had just said.

"Couple weeks. I'll do it in my office."

"What about the drain?"

"Before you're discharged."

"And when will that be?"

"Soon as possible. Four, five days."

Doctor Pettle turned to face Doctor Blatt. "What were his latest sed rate and CRP results?"

"Not back from the lab yet. Should know later today."

"Can you give the nurses permission to give me test results directly? I'd hate to pester you with questions."

"Sure, that's fine."

"Wonderful. Thank you again for your splendid work, Doctor."

This seemed to lighten Doctor Blatt's mood, to elevate him. "Of course. I'm really very happy with how it's turned out so far. Still a long way to go, of course. I'm hoping we'll be able to save that leg in the long run."

"As am I. As are we all. Well, thank you again."

Doctor Blatt nodded and turned to leave, bloated with pride, unaware that he had just been dismissed from the room.

"Not the best bedside manner, that's for sure," Doctor Pettle said once he was gone. "But his work is impeccable."

"You think so?" Deirdre asked.

"Well, without seeing the bone and implant, it's hard to say for sure. But from the looks of things, he's tidied it all up remarkably. And the fact that you've been able to get up and about so quickly, Patrick—I know it must be frustrating, how slow it goes, but it is truly remarkable given where you were before."

That night, and for the remainder of his stay, Deirdre slept at Patrick's apartment. She wouldn't have admitted it, but the cramped quarters of the hospital room—especially sleeping in that chair—were beginning to take their toll, not just physically, but on her whole person. She needed the world to seem larger, more spacious and full. She needed this not only for herself but also for Patrick, needed to be able to remind him, to enact in subtle ways, the broad and enlivening complexity of things outside and beyond this place. Each night, after dinner, she would silently start moving around the room, arranging things neatly, closing up for the day. She would tuck him in, lingering over every fold in the sheets, before leaning to kiss his forehead and saying goodnight. And then—almost calmly, but not quite—she would drape her light coat around her, turn down the lights, and head out. And once back at the flat, she slept recklessly, throwing herself fully into the rest, her body absorbing the sleep as if it were stocking its larders for a brutal wintertide.

36

The second time he went home was easier than the time before. He steeled himself against the transition by anticipating its rough and compassionless edges, knowing full well that the first few days would be the worst. Doctor Pettle helped, writing prescriptions for the medications he needed a day in advance, ensuring that the pain at least would be held at bay. Deirdre braced herself, too, preparing the space of the flat to resemble, as closely as she could imagine, his home before everything had begun. She placed photographs on tables and counters and, in homage to his relative untidiness, scattered a few books around here and there.

On the day of his departure, Patrick was pushed through the roughest of his physical therapy trainings yet: ascending and descending stairs. For this schooling he was rewarded with a pair of old wooden crutches, the walker holding too much depth and girth for an average step. Marcus was helping him now, standing in the hallway before a wooden prop of a staircase, four levels up.

"You're going to have to rely on your upper-body strength for this. But don't forget your balance. You're out of practice, and your body might not remember what it feels like to right itself. Just be aware of where you are in the process."

"What if I fall?"

"I'm ready to catch you. Try not to think about it. Just focus on taking baby steps, feeling the shift of your weight forward and back, side to side."

"OK, OK. I'm ready."

"Good leg first, then the crutches, then the bad, OK? Get all your weight steadied on the crutches before bringing the left leg up."

Patrick positioned the crutches on the floor, adjusting their feet meticulously so that they were evenly lined up. He paused, focusing on the feel of his soles on the ground, sensing the difference in pressure between the right and the left.

"Remember, the crutches are standing in for your left leg. Let them do their job. Push into them with your arms. Ready?"

"I think so." Patrick stretched his right leg up to the plain of the bottom stair, placed it exactly in the middle. He felt a slow twist of pain, nothing serious or severe, more like soreness—then reached the crutches up and began pushing with all his might, through the arms, down towards the floor. Heaving a great breath, he swung his left leg up, planting it down next to the right.

"Woah!" he said, looking around. He could see the top of Marcus's head now, noticed a slight balding pattern near its peak. "Ha! I did it!"

"Good job, Patrick. Feel steady?"

"Yes! Easy!" A small trickle of sweat began to make its way from his hairline down to his ear.

"Steady now, let's go for number two."

"OK. OK. Here we go." He repeated the procedure, tipping slightly to the left, Marcus securing him at the last moment.

"Alright, take a rest before the next one."

"No, I want to keep going. I want to get to the top. While I've got some momentum."

"OK, but easy now …" Marcus began to grip his upper arms, holding him in place.

He took the last steps in quick succession, swinging himself from one to the next with a regular rhythm. Once at the top he laughed, looking around, noticing how different the hall looked from here. He could see the dusty top edges of picture frames, and the floor behind the nurses' desk, previously hidden from his usual perspective. He beamed at the hall and everyone in it, and was rewarded with a small bit of applause from a nurse nearby, a thumbs-up from another patient huddling past, dragging her IV rack beside her.

"OK?" Marcus asked. "Ready to descend?"

"Give me a minute," Patrick said, "to enjoy the view." He held his position, craning his head around in both directions, one after the other. Deirdre stood twenty feet away, smiling at him. "OK, let's do it," he finally said.

"Good. First, pivot in place so you're facing the other direction, just like we practiced. First the crutches, then your feet. Remember your balance."

Patrick did as he was told, then froze in place: the descent suddenly seemed terrifying. "Woah," he said. "This is worse than going up."

"Yep, that's right. More accidents happen going down than going up."

"What do I do?"

"Focus only on the step right in front of you. Forget the rest. Deirdre? Deirdre—I want you to come watch this closely. You'll be helping when he does this outside." She walked over tenderly, not wanting to interrupt. She had her book open, writing everything down. "OK, now you work in reverse: first the crutches to the lower step, holding your weight on your good leg. Once they're steady, move the bad leg down—"

"Wait," Patrick said. "Stop."

Marcus looked up, "Want me to start over?"

"No, no—I'm with you. But can we *not* call it my 'bad' leg? It hasn't done anything wrong. It doesn't want this any more than I do."

"Yes, sure. Of course. Your *left* leg. First the crutches, then your *left* leg. Once they're all in place, press hard into the crutches and bring your right leg down. Focus on balance, OK?"

"OK."

"Deirdre, your job is to move with him, in front of him, down every step. You'll need to get used to bracing yourself; he's so much taller than you. If he starts to get uneasy, *do not* try to steady the crutches. Don't even touch them, OK? Let them fall if they fall. Your job is to steady *him*. Be ready to catch him around the waist if something goes wrong. Got it?"

"Got it."

"Watch me while he comes down. Ready, Patrick?"

"Ready."

They moved steadily as a team, in unison, Marcus always a step below Patrick, focused intently on his midsection, from his center of gravity down to his waist. Patrick reached, stepped, reached, stepped, taking small breaks between each stage of descent. His arms quivered slightly at first, but had stopped by the time they were halfway down.

"Great! Great. First try. Really great job, Patrick."

"Oof," Patrick said. "That's not easy."

"Well you sure made it *look* easy. Deirdre, you ready to try your part? Why don't you spot him in both directions, up and down. I'll need to see you do it at least twice before I can sign off on the discharge."

And so it went, each step a simple victory; each pass of the stairs a minor performance, opening night, full house, ovation not quite standing but an ovation nonetheless.

An hour before, Marcus had removed the drain. This was, as Patrick had learned, one of the strangest, if simplest, procedures of the whole. Pulling the dressing back, Marcus said, "Ready? I'm about to pull," while pressing down over the wound with his left hand. He grasped the bottom of the tube with his right, at just the point where it entered him, and then suddenly dragged it out in one big, broad move. The tube flopped and dripped, protesting its rude awakening with a sound like slurping: messy, childish, course.

The pulling itself felt sexual. There is no other way to describe it: the wound was briefly converted into an erogenous zone, one whose sensations stopped just before pleasure, a point of strange two-ness that offered no finishing shock of implosion, no final release. It *did* send strong shudders, a systemic tremble, up and down Patrick's spine, making of his whole person a tingling, vibrating thing.

He was always bashful when it was done, blushing as he looked at the nurse performing the removal—in this case, Marcus. He always wondered if the nurse knew what this felt like, had felt it before, precisely because it was so intimate, so erotic, so overwhelmingly (if briefly) obscene. And then the wound would begin to itch, jarring him out of the blush, bringing him up from the reverie, waking him up.

"Huh," he breathed, light-headed and dazed. "Whoosh, just like that."

"All done," Marcus said, dropping the tube in a bin. "Good?"

"Glad it's out," he replied, turning away. "Whoosh." He wondered again if Marcus knew how it felt, or could read it on his face. He turned further away, tucking his head deeper into the pillow, and closed his eyes. "Whoosh," drawn out like a long-building sough.

"Keep the leg dry. No showers or baths." Doctor Blatt was standing next to the bed, eyes on the clipboard and papers he held. "Home care will help with the antibiotics and will run regular tests like before. You've got an appointment for a couple weeks from now, my office, where I'll remove the staples. Come back again a couple weeks after that."

Maria was tending to the wound, redressing it for travel. She secured the last piece of tape in place and smoothed out the gauze. "That feel OK?" she asked. "Not too tight?"

"Good, thanks," Patrick told her. He gave her a subtle smile and, at the last moment, a small wink. She winked back.

Deirdre was rummaging through a bag, making sure she had the keys. "Thank you, Doctor Blatt," she said.

"Get up and move, Patrick, as much as you can. But not too much weight on that leg. OK?"

"OK."

"Good. Well. That's all for now. Good luck. See you soon."

"See you soon."

Maria reached over and squeezed his arm. "See you very soon," she said, and gave him another wink.

Up out of bed, he scooted the walker ahead of him, following Marcus out into the hall. His clothes felt strange on him, too clingy when compared to the gown; and his shoes—even the clogs his mother had brought, loose enough to fit around the swelling—were tight, constricting. He jimmied his toes up and down, back-and-forth as often as he could while stepping. "I can't just use the crutches?" he asked Marcus. "They're more age-appropriate."

"Best if you don't. You need more support for now."

"This thing is embarrassing."

"Why?"

Patrick looked up at him. "What?"

"Why is it embarrassing?"

"I don't know—it just feels old, rickety. Makes *me* feel old and rickety, too. Makes me feel like people are staring at me. Conspicuous."

"A lot of people use walkers."

"Yeah, but ..." he looked at the floor.

"Yeah, but what?"

"Not people like me."

"And what does *that* mean? What are *people like you*?" He seemed vaguely offended.

"Too young for a walker."

Marcus sighed and placed his hands on the walker, stopping Patrick's forward motion. "Look, I've never had to use one of these things myself, OK? So I don't really know what it feels like. But I *can* tell you that a lot of people come through these rooms. And they're lucky to get out, whether it's in a chair or on a walker or with crutches—they're lucky to get out."

"So you're telling me to keep my chin up, something like that."

"I guess I am, yes." He was staring Patrick down now, refusing to loosen his glare. "Chin up. You can do this. I don't care what Doctor Blatt says. You can get through this. *With* your leg—*both* good legs. You'll walk again."

"You think so?"

"I do. You will walk again. But only if you take it slowly, measure out each stage in the process and go through it slowly, properly. The walker is one of the stages."

"So I have to *earn* the crutches?"

"Damn straight."

Patrick snorted and smirked, not quite convinced. "Fine. OK. I'll shut up about the walker."

Marcus let go and backed away. "Good. So you're going to walk out of here, right? Don't want the wheelchair for the ride down?"

"Damn straight," Patrick said. "I want to walk."

As he moved down the hall, eyes on the elevator, focused intensely on shifting and stepping as Marcus had taught him, he became aware that he *was* being watched: by the others on this hall, not yet well enough to leave. A woman with sharp eyes and matted hair followed him most of the way, pulling her IV rack with her as she moved, advising him of obstacles in the way. "Bunch of chairs coming up," she said, "sticking out on the left." One man, heavy and bent, mumbled encouragement: "You *go*, son. You *go* with your bad self. *Get* that walking, now, *get* it." A child, couldn't have been more than twelve, bald, skin alit with the excitement of some recent treatment, smiled and waved the whole way. Patrick waved back, in one final gesture, as the elevator doors shuddered and closed.

37

Deirdre sat on the couch, her legs tucked up underneath her. She was on the phone, waiting again on another hold. Papers were scattered next to her, strewn across the cushions almost all the way to the opposite side. She held two of them, inspecting them, trying to make sense.

"Yes, hello. I'm still here," she suddenly said. "No, please, don't put me on hold again." She paused, listened, then sighed and closed her eyes. "I don't understand how these people can just *do* this," she said. "I've been on the phone for an hour."

Patrick was sitting in the easy chair, looking through stacks of bills. "A hundred dollars for a pill? This is bizarre. I mean, they list it all out—*everything*. Twenty dollars for a nutritional shake. Is this even legal?"

"I don't know, Patrick."

"Four thousand, five hundred, sixty dollars for anesthesia? For a single surgery?" He shifted to another page. "One thousand, four hundred, eighty-four dollars for lab tests? Two thousand, seven hundred, sixty-eight dollars for the spinal tap? It took *five minutes*." He turned to a third page. "Oh my God. Fourteen thousand dollars for an MRI." He scanned the columns and rows. "Look at this! They charge for each thing they want to look at, each different part of the spine and hip. Between a thousand and twenty-five hundred dollars a pop. They *can't* be serious. And here's another one, from a week later. Same MRIs, same areas. Sixteen thousand."

"Yes, I'm still here," Deirdre said into the phone. "No, please—don't ..."

"These numbers are out of control. How do they *do* this?" He began scanning the sheets, looking for any kind of relief from their strange, opaque calculus. "What's an *adjustment*?"

"I think that's an insurance thing. They waive part of the cost, some kind of agreement with the insurance company."

"So if you have insurance, everything costs less?"

"I don't know. I guess so."

"And if you don't have insurance, everything costs more?"

"I don't know, Patrick."

"How does that even make *sense*?"

"Hello? Yes, hello. Please don't put me on hold again. I've been on the phone for an hour." Deirdre sat up, finally getting some attention. "I'm calling about my son's claims. He's been in and out of the hospital. We've been getting notices about the lifetime limit.... Yes, he's right here. Hang on." She handed Patrick the phone. "They need to talk to you."

"Hello? Yes, this is Patrick." He listened to a thin voice on the other end, conscious of its impatience. "Yes, thank you. My mom is trying to sort all of this out. Can you talk to her?"

"We need your approval first."

"OK, I approve. Is that what you need me to say?"

"Well, technically we need you to sign a form first. But I can grant access for this phone call only based on your verbal approval. I'll just need to record you first. You'll hear a click, then a beep. When you hear that, state your full name and social security number, then give the full name of the person you're allowing us to talk to, OK?"

"Sure, OK." Patrick did as instructed, then handed the phone back to Deirdre.

"Hello? Are you there? Good, OK. So we got these notices about the lifetime limit. We don't know what they mean." She went quiet, listening closely, taking notes. "And how much is left?" She went quiet again, a deeper silence, registering what she was told. "Eighty percent? Are you sure?" She jotted something down, doubling over the numbers and lines, etching them in. "What about the bills we keep getting? From the hospital? They say he owes thousands of dollars. Why isn't all of this stuff covered?" She waited again.

Patrick began to feel as if he were sinking, the bills like quicksand around him. "*Sixteen thousand dollars,*" he murmured to himself. "Sixteen thousand. Just like that."

"But some of the statements from you say 'Patient Responsibility, zero.' For the same dates of service, same hospital, same stuff. What does that mean?" She kept writing.

He imagined himself skimming along an ocean of bills, trying to surf over them but constantly pulled down. He thought how trite that feeling must be, how common. He considered writing it down, just to mark its banality as a cliché. Buried in bills, sinking in bills, swallowed by bills. He thought of these metaphors, these explanations of a general feeling of being overwhelmed by obligation, of not being able to make the ends meet. How simple they were, how concise and how true. He looked over at Deirdre, who was wearing one of her panicked looks, trying not to let it show.

"And for the last twenty percent, do you know how long it will last? Will it cover the last two surgeries? ... No, of course not, I'm sorry, I know you can't predict. But if the last two cost the same as the first, I mean the first of this kind, how long will it last? The last twenty percent.... Yes, he's getting home care now. For the next six weeks.... Yes, a lot of prescriptions." She put down her pen. "OK. OK." She thought for a moment. "Who do we talk to about increasing the lifetime maximum? ... *Who* did that? *Berkeley*? ... I see. OK. OK, thank you." She put the phone down, looked at her book, and then closed it and put it aside.

Patrick had the feeling that he did not need to ask how the conversation had gone. He could piece things together on his own, having heard only Deirdre's side. He started stacking the pages on his lap together, tamping them into a neat pile, and handed them to Deirdre. "I don't think I can keep working on this right now."

"Me either," she said. "Let's look at them again tomorrow. Maybe get Tim or Doctor Pettle to help." She began cleaning up, organizing everything into its place, into its proper folder and file. She had bought a small box for these things, which was already beginning to overflow.

After lunch, Deirdre began packing Patrick up and getting him ready for a new round of appointments, these with the ophthalmologist who would begin working on the damage to Patrick's retinas. They had put this off for too long, but it had been a necessary delay: there had simply been no time to deal with eyes and leg together, no energy for the constant transporting, no space beyond the pain in the bones that had summoned them into its all-encompassing command.

"It's really endless, isn't it," Patrick said lazily. "I mean, this is my entire life. One doctor after another. Bills. Confusion, sitting around. This is it. This is everything."

"I thought we might drive around the lake when we're done. Maybe even get out, go sit on a bench. People-watch."

"OK."

"Maybe see if Robin—or Fergus, or Jan, or maybe Kevin—want to meet us for dinner? At that burger place you like?"

"Sure. Sounds good."

She sat down in the middle of her preparation, squared off to face him. "You know, I do need to go home for a little while. Back east. Just to get settled a bit, get some things done."

Patrick looked at his lap. "Yeah. I figured you might."

"I'd like to start bringing some of your friends in more, get them into the swing of helping out. So it won't be so hard on you when I'm gone."

"Yeah."

"Kevin said he and Ronaldo could spend the night the day I leave. Jan the night after that. And then Robin. What do you think about that?"

"Probably a good idea, at least for a few nights." He looked up at her. "I *am* pretty nervous." He began rubbing his hands together, slowly but firmly, working something out. "I mean, I know you need to go. It'll be good for you. And for me. But I'm nervous about it. I'm so dependent."

"Great thing about your friends, Patrick: they really want to help. It's been kind of amazing, actually, how insistent they are. They're just waiting for you to give the word."

"I know."

"You have some great friends, really, really great. I never knew that about you, never knew just how close you were to so many people."

"They're family," Patrick said, "not just friends."

"I can tell."

"My siblings, my kin."

"I've never seen anything like it. Camped out in the waiting room. Calling me to check on you *and* me. Offering to bring food. Constantly, since this all began."

"They're family."

"Yep." She stood up and walked to him, "Ready to go?"

"Yeah. Hey, when do you think you should head back?"

"Couple days."

"Have you looked at tickets?"

"Yes."

"Go ahead and get one. Maybe call while I'm in this appointment. Get it settled. It'll help me to know what to expect, and when."

"Alright. I will." She brought him the walker, helped him slowly rise to meet it, then left him to maneuver himself over to the door. He was solid on his feet now, moving with speed, seeming not even to notice the apparatus that enabled him to walk.

"Maybe we should try the crutches," he said once he'd gotten just outside the door.

"Maybe we should. Let's try when we get back tonight, OK? I don't want to push it."

"Yeah, OK," he said, pivoting in place and then moving prudently towards the stairs.

Doctor Straddler was tall, almost six-four, and lanky; but he moved gracefully, like a dancer, conscious of the breadth stretched by his limbs. His office was on the fourth floor of a heritage building in Oakland, sharp red brick bordered by ornate plaster crests and other figures who stared down at the sidewalk ominously, as they had done for nearly 100 years. Inside, the building was pristine in its recent renovations; but the great expense of updating it had been spent on a modest design, resulting in a clean, usable interior that was equal parts efficiency and warmth. The elevator had not been replaced, and was beautiful—if slow and cantankerous—in its distinctly pre-modern style. It had an iron gate, which had to be pulled shut and wrenched open again at the appropriate points in the process of ascending and descending floors. There was even a stool in its corner, built into its walls, where a man had once sat to accompany visitors up and down. Of all the lifts he had ridden over the past few months, this was Patrick's favorite, even though it sometimes felt as if its cables might snap, tired from years of work, and drop the box straight down to the sub-basement floor.

"*You've* come a long way," Doctor Straddler said once Patrick was in the chair.

"Have I?"

"Oh yeah. Hard to believe you're the same person from months ago, when you were still in and out." He had been in the room that third time Patrick had awoken, so long ago, operating the machines pointed at his eyes, inserting the needles. "But here you are. On the mend. How are those eyes?"

"I guess they seem stable. I'm still getting used to them, the way they are now."

"Well, they're still damn good eyes, Patrick. You'll get used to them eventually." He used a small magnifying glass and a flashlight to test the pupils, gauge their response rates. "You know, we're learning more and more that we 'see' with our brains, not with the eyes themselves. Even when there's been this much damage, the brain works to piece images together, making sense of the visual world."

"I kind of get that," Patrick said. "It's weird—when I'm looking out at the world, just an ordinary scene, the blank spots sort of fizzle and fade; they stop appearing as just big black holes. Sometimes they look like static on a television. When I look towards something that's flat and plain, like a wall, or a sky without clouds, they disappear entirely—so it looks like itself, whatever it is, the wall, the sky. Like it always has. Without the spots."

"That's right. That's the brain at work."

"What is it doing? The brain I mean. How is it working?"

"Well, it gathers whatever visual information is available, then fills in the holes. So when you're looking at an empty wall, say, the brain will take color and shading information from the area around the blank spots, and then fills them in, making the image whole."

"Huh," Patrick said. "Amazing."

"It really is. Of course, the brain can't do everything—if you're looking at an irregular field, something complex, the brain doesn't know *what* is behind the blank spots. So it has to guess, based on what other things have looked like before."

"Really?"

"Oh yes. It has all this visual information stored, like a vast library of images. It knows how typical something is in your experience, how common a particular image might be. And it uses that information to fill in the gaps." He had Patrick's head back now, administering drops to dilate the pupils. "Sometimes that can lead to strange mistakes, things seeming to appear out of nowhere. Things that aren't really there."

"That's happened once or twice, like a hallucination—I wasn't sure *what* was going on."

"Has it? When?"

"Like the other day. We were out somewhere, I can't remember, I think on our way to get lunch. I was looking around the sidewalk, and I thought I saw my grandmother there suddenly, smiling at me. But of course she wasn't. I assumed I'd just seen someone who looked like her, but I didn't: there was only a kid and his mom, walking in the opposite direction."

"Interesting."

"So you think my *brain* did that?"

"Possibly, yes. Maybe you'd been in a similar place before, or multiple times before; or maybe you were thinking of your grandmother unconsciously. So your brain might have expected her to be there, and then pulled up an image of her to fill in the blank spot."

"That has got to be one of the most incredible things I've ever heard."

"Vision is incredibly complex. Wrapped up with all sorts of other things: memories, dreams, desires, fears. It pulls in all these other aspects of your mental and emotional life, of your present and past, of what you want for the future. Pulls them all in to make an image."

"Even for people with regular vision?"

"Yes, even for us." Doctor Straddler pulled Patrick's right eyelid back, holding open the eye to get a full view of its interior. "But we don't get a sense of that, those of us who haven't been through what you have. We might never know how complicated vision is, how subjective it is. We take it for granted, in more ways than one. Assume it's just base reality, nothing more than a reflection of fact. Nothing could be further from the truth."

Patrick thought about this, marveling through it, while the doctor shifted to his left eye, repeated the inspection there.

"In other words, Patrick, you're getting a rigorous sense of what vision really *is*. A rare, really rare, sense of it." He paused, concentrating on something deep inside. "Have you noticed any changes here? In the left eye—near the periphery of your visual field."

"A little bit of flickering from time to time. Almost like a blinking light. And—oh, right, I forgot about this—in the hospital, the day before I was discharged this last time, I saw larger flashes, like blue lightning."

"Blue lightning?"

"Kind of. Not really lightning bolts. But moving lines of blue light, from top to bottom, then back-and-forth across the middle."

"Interesting. Any changes in the vision itself after that?"

"Well, I don't want to say this—I know you've said there's no way to fix things in there. But it did seem to get sharper, more detailed, after that. And one of the spots seemed to get just a little bit smaller. Not much. I'm not even sure it really happened. Why?"

"It's healing very nicely, the left eye. There's a spot to the extreme side of the retina—I was worried about it before, not sure it would dry out the way it should, thought it might leave a wrinkle, creating pressure on the retina as a whole. That would put you at risk for more damage, another tear."

"And now?"

"It has calmed down, settled back into place. The swelling seems to be down. We'll do an angiogram just to be sure. But I think you may have been seeing it heal; the light you saw may have been a mixture of inflammation and then healing."

"So good news, right?"

"Oh yeah. Very good news." He straightened Patrick's chair, upright again, then put his tools away and pulled up a stool. "There are still some places of concern in the right eye. It would be hard for you to notice them; so many changes, and your visual field is so much smaller in that eye—really, limited to the peripheries on three sides. We'll do the angiogram, check for leakage from the capillaries there. I may need to do another laser surgery to stop them from growing, if indeed there is a problem. That would result in more, or larger, blank spots."

"So bad news, too."

"A little. But it's not really something you'll notice, not too much anyway, given that it's in your right eye. The left eye looks good, solid, stable." He gave this a moment to sink in, then asked: "How well are you reading?"

"Pretty well, I guess. Slower than before."

"And moving around? Do you bump into things?"

"Not so much. With the left eye I can make out most everything now. Much better than when this started, I mean. I can see people again, and faces. The spots are annoying—but like I said, I'm getting used to them."

"Good."

"Do you ..." he paused for a moment. "Do you think I'll be able to drive again?"

"I do, actually. I do. But let's not get ahead of ourselves, OK? Let's make sure everything here is settled first. Let's start with the angiogram, in the next room over."

"OK. Yes, OK." He started to pull himself forward, out of the chair. He wasn't sure, but he thought he started to feel a spring in his step, a slight bounce, a hint of weightlessness, as he followed the doctor out of the room, skin alive and electric, eyes full and wide, and his lips turned up in the most subtle of all arcs, hope wafting forward and out from him like too much jasmine perfume.

38

Days stretched out before him; he was able to count them, marking the move forward towards the next surgery, and ultimately towards the last. He had begun to plan it all out in his head, pacing himself, like a long-distance run.

"Your sed rate, Patrick, is back in normal range. And the best part is, it's stayed there. Over a month." Doctor Pettle looked over at him, beaming, genuinely pleased. "This is the best possible news. Just great."

"So the infection is gone?"

"Probably not yet gone entirely. But it is completely controlled."

"Like a wildfire, ninety percent contained."

"Ha-ha, yes, that's right. Ninety percent contained."

"But still burning."

"Probably smoldering. But contained. That's the key part."

Patrick smiled, too. It was an accomplishment, he felt, one that had not come easily—not for him or anyone else. Illness was a team sport, he thought, and everyone involved deserved the win.

"How's Deirdre doing? She's been back home, what, a week now?"

"Just under a week. She seems good, probably feeling guilty not to be here, but glad to be home for a break."

"And you? Are you managing alone?"

"I am absolutely *not* managing alone. I have you, and Thuy every other day, and a long list of friends who take turns spending the night, bringing me food. Tonight it's Kevin and Ronaldo again. They're making pork chops."

"What great friends you have. And your neighbors seem nice."

"Oh—yes. Bobbi and Charlotte, first apartment down near the stairs. Both psychiatric nurses at General. They check on me every day, take me down to their place to hang out. They're hilarious. Bobbi said she'd cut my hair when I want it."

"And—what's her name, next door?"

"Jez."

"Yes, Jez. She stopped me on my way up. Asked who I was, why I was bothering you."

"Ha-ha, yeah, she's my guardian. She's stuck at home right now too, back problems. Keeps her windows open to keep an eye out for any invaders. Sometimes I watch talk shows with her, during the day. She's taking me to my eye appointment next week."

"Great building you live in. People watching out for each other."

"And I didn't even really know them that well before, just knew their names."

"Strangers have a way of coming together when there's crisis. So, sounds like you're well taken care of. Any bases not covered? Anything you feel that you need?"

"Well, these bills ... and the insurance company. I don't know, there's probably nothing anyone can do. But they keep coming, so many overdue. Huge amounts, too, especially when you add them all up."

"How much?"

"Last count, something like thirty-five, forty thousand. But they're still catching up, haven't gotten much from the last hospital stay yet. Plus home care. I don't know, I mean, there's really nothing I can do. I don't know what they expect. How many people have that kind of money just lying around? Even people *with* health insurance."

"Yes—it's really very tragic."

"I can't imagine what it would be like *not* to have coverage. I mean, even those numbers: they include huge adjustments, discounts worked out with the insurance company. I'd owe three or four times that if I didn't have insurance, if I was truly poor."

"It's one of the great ironies of our failed system. Hospitals survive by charging exorbitant amounts, especially to people who can't pay. And then eventually, they just write it all off—a tax break, and in order to stay solvent they need to write off as much as possible. That's why the costs are lower for people with insurance. Because people with insurance can actually *pay*."

"That sounds like the most backwards system anyone could possibly imagine."

"It is."

"So people without insurance have to declare bankruptcy, right? So the hospital can get the write-off."

"Usually, yes. Sometimes the hospital will just write it off themselves, zeroing out the balance."

"How do I get them to do that for *me*?"

"I wouldn't do anything, not yet, if I were you. Wait until all is said and done, after the last surgery. Just stay in touch with the accounts people. Let them know you're still in and out of the hospital."

"Then what?"

"Best I can say, just keep calling, keep writing letters. Let them know you're a student, will soon be a teacher. There's no way you can pay these bills. Beg for their mercy. Beg them to write off as much as they can."

"Will that work?"

"Honestly, I have no idea. I've never seen it work, not smoothly or without a struggle at least. Most people just declare bankruptcy in this situation."

Patrick looked at him. "I can't believe that's how this all works."

"It is not," Doctor Pettle said, "the most humane system imaginable. To say the least."

Patrick thought of those people, the countless legions of them, who had no mother sifting assiduously through paperwork, no network of friends to bring food, no doctors who'd taken such close care. He shook his head, closed his eyes.

"I just cannot believe that this is how it works," he said. "All those people. My God. All those people with no one to help."

Tugboat Tim dropped by at four, done with work for the day.

"Hey, whatever happened with that project? The test? With the ship?" Patrick asked him.

"Oh—that. It worked out, eventually. Took us a couple tries, but we figured out how to maneuver."

"So Marin is saved."

"Marin will be fine." Tim smiled at him.

"But not Oakland."

"Oakland'll be fine, too. We worked it out."

"Phew," Patrick said.

"Your mom called me today. She sounds good. Wanted to make sure you were doing OK."

"What'd you tell her?"

"That you were better than OK. I don't think she believed me."

"She doesn't believe me, either," Patrick said, both of them laughing.

"Hey, listen. About the other day."

Two days before, Tim had shown up with a gleam in his eye, which Patrick returned. They had nestled for a while on the couch, then moved precipitously to the bedroom, Tim carrying Patrick so he wouldn't need the crutches or walker. It had rained that day, heavy and loud, a strong wind pushing against the windows—which had struck them both as a perfect accompaniment to what they were up to.

"Yeah?" Patrick said.

"It was fun. For you, too?"

"For me, too."

"Felt good." Nothing too intense or involved had happened; but things had progressed, as they are wont to do, beyond everyday intimacy—unless your everyday is especially charged. "Felt very good."

"Yeah. It did. I'd forgotten what it felt like to be in my body like that, to be *with* someone who isn't, you know, operating on me."

"Ha-ha. I can imagine. Well, no, I can't. Anyway, listen. I didn't want to mention it before, didn't want to get you worried. Just wanted to enjoy it, especially falling asleep next to you afterwards. But … well, listen, when you finished, there was some blood."

"Some blood? Where?"

"You know, when you *finished*." He looked at Patrick with cheeky eyes, giving special emphasis to the final word, drawing it out.

"Oh. *Oh.* I see. Yes. OK. They said that could happen."

"Who did?"

"Doctor Pettle—and Diana once, a while ago."

"They said there might be blood?"

"Yes. They told me it's nothing to worry about, not unless there's a lot of it, or it doesn't stop."

"Ah. OK. Wow, OK. Huh." He seemed to relax suddenly, like he had been carrying something on his back, something that had just vanished, dissipating into the air. He leaned back, slinging an arm around Patrick's shoulders. "Whew."

Patrick smirked, "Have you been worried about it?"

"Well, *yes*, obviously, I've been worried about it. I wasn't sure what to do, just cleaned it up before you saw. Didn't want to mention it right away, like I said. But it's been on my mind. Whew!" Tim rolled his eyes, an exaggerated gesture of relief. He turned and grinned, "OK, good. Glad we got that out of the way."

"Me, too. But do me a favor, OK? Don't hang on to things like that. I don't want you to worry. And I can handle it, really. I can handle it."

"OK."

"Promise?"

"Promise."

He really *could* handle it, he thought. But something else began to rise in him, a caution, an embarrassment, some shame. That such a moment, such a series of charged moments, could be permeated by anything close to distaste, especially when held in reserve, kept back, kept secret—it tarred the event, that momentous event, stripped it of its momentousness, wrote it back into the story that he was so desperate to draw to a close.

"I know what you're thinking," Tim said out of the blue.

"You do?"

"Yeah, I do." Patrick believed that he did. "Stop thinking it. Right now. Stop thinking it." Tim pulled him closer, a profoundly deep and decisive embrace. And Patrick tried, he really tried, to stop thinking—but it was done, it was already thought, and the best he could do was to stop remembering, to cast that day back into a blur of other days, and enjoy the feel of what was right in front of and around him: that distinctive sensation of two arms that do not belong to you wrapped around your whole body, making you theirs.

"Suzanne, beware of the devil," he began to sing softly. "Don't let him spoil your heart."

Tim squeezed harder, pulled him in. "I hope you're not singing about me."

Doctor Blatt's office was really a clinic, arranged compactly in a ground-floor wing of one of the hospital's clustered buildings. For an orthopedic unit, it was remarkably difficult to get into: too many doors, too many angles to maneuver oneself through and around. The waiting room was laid out like betting windows at the tracks: long and narrow, with chairs and banquettes lining the walls. A central desk rose up high in the very middle of the room, the staff working there surrounded on all sides. When Patrick arrived at the desk to check in, the woman said: "Get comfortable."

"I'm sorry?"

"Get comfortable."

"Oh, I'm not *that* early. My appointment's in ten minutes."

The woman looked up at him. "This your first time here?" she asked.

"Yes."

"Doctor's running late. About two hours."

"Two *hours*?"

"Two hours."

"Should I leave and come back?"

"Only if you want to risk losing your appointment."

"Oh. OK. Is there somewhere I could sit? No chairs out here. And I can't really stand with this thing the whole time," he said, nodding down to the walker.

The woman looked at him, confused, then stood up and looked down; she hadn't seen, before, that he was using it, assumed he was just another kid with a twist or sprain. "Oh, honey," she said, "I'm sorry. I didn't see. Hold on, let me come around." Tim came in just then, having dropped Patrick off and parked the car in the garage.

Standing next to him now, the woman looked around the room. "Listen up, people. These chairs are for patients. I see a lot of family members sitting down. I need somebody to move—*now*—to make space for this young man.... You know the rules, now come on, somebody, *up*." Nobody moved, except to avert their eyes, hoping they wouldn't be seen. "You, right there, sir, you a patient?" She pointed to a robust-looking blond man, big biceps and legs, who was studiously reading an old issue of *Sports Illustrated*. "Hey, *you*," she said, walking closer and pointing.

The man jerked his head up. "Me? What?"

"You a patient or a family member?"

"I'm here with my mother." He pointed at someone across the room.

"Get up."

"Excuse me?"

"Get *up*." She tilted her head to gesture to Patrick. "He needs a seat."

The man looked astonished, as if this request was going too far; as if she would be sorry for disturbing him; as if her boss would hear about this, just wait. And so on. He stood up begrudgingly, and made a sweeping, sardonic gesture with his arm before walking away in a huff.

"This work OK?" she asked Patrick.

"It's fine, thank you. Thank you so much." He turned around gingerly and lowered himself into the seat.

"OK. Fill these out and give them back to me." She handed him a stack of papers, fixed precariously to a clipboard. They were the usual set of intake forms, name, address, insurance information; then medical history with boxes in rows; and then pain information: the ten-point scale, the outline of a human body with space for him to indicate its location. He filled them out neatly and precisely within two minutes, barely thinking as he went down the list. Tim stood to the side, squeezed between the chair and a small side table, stacked messily with outdated magazines. A fluorescent bulb flickered in the fixture above his head; he looked up at it, wondering if he could reach up and jostle it into place.

"Want a Coke?" he asked Patrick. "I saw a machine in the hall."

"No thanks."

Time dripped by, water oozing from a leaky faucet. Occasionally someone's name was called; they would rouse themselves up from where they were perched and slowly lumber to the doors at the back of the room, where someone else was waiting to take them in.

Patrick was watching an older woman sitting across from him. She sat slumped in her chair, next to a young boy holding her bags. She stared into the space before her, eyes fogged and unfocused. Her legs seemed twisted and worn, unevenly spaced on the floor in front of her. The left one pointed at an impractical angle, too far inward. She heaved great sighs as she sat, each one seeming to deflate her further. Patrick felt great heaviness as he looked at her, as if he was watching a version of himself in fifty years. He could sense that she was in pain, could feel that she had gotten used to it, forgetting what it was like not to bear it. When her name was called, it took a good five minutes for her to stand and move carefully over to the doors.

Tim watched Patrick's looking. When the woman had finally left the room, he reached down and put his hand on Patrick's shoulder. "That's not you, you know." He smiled faintly as he caught Patrick's eye.

"I know. But it's not that far off, either."

"Farther off than you think."

After a little more than an hour, the woman from the desk came over and leaned down. "I was able to squeeze you in a little early. They'll be calling you in soon, OK?"

"OK," Patrick said. The pain meds were beginning to wear off; and because he had thought this would be an in-and-out affair, he had not brought any more with him. His body ached, the beginning stages of a full throbbing return.

"You look uncomfortable."

"Pain's coming back."

"Why don't you go ahead and get up, move around a little. Might help work some of it out."

Tim pulled the walker back into place; Patrick rose slowly, deliberately, and then took a few steps away from the chair. The ache subsided slightly, dissipating from his hip and releasing down the leg. He lightened, straightening himself, looking up and around. "Better," he said.

In the exam room, he changed into a gown and then was hoisted by Tim up onto the bed, covered in clean rolled paper. It sounded like dry autumn leaves being swept to a pile. He wiggled back into place, his legs dangling off the end.

Doctor Blatt and Maria rushed in, clearly in the middle of a long day, endless appointments like this one.

"Sorry for the wait," he said. "We had a trauma case come into the ER this morning, and everything got backed up. How's that leg?" Maria busied herself with his paperwork, spending most of her time reading the page on pain.

"Much better than before. Still some aches, but it doesn't feel as heavy or full. Hard to explain. And I've been able to sleep through the night again."

"Good. Let's take a look."

Patrick pulled himself back further onto the bed until his legs were stretched straight out in front of him. The doctor grabbed his left shin, twisting it slightly inward, then out.

"Feel this?"

"Yes."

He traced lines on the bottom of Patrick's foot with his index finger. "How about this?"

"Yep."

"Good." He reached and lifted the base of the gown, exposing the long bandage on top of the scar. He picked at its edges, then pulled it away in one long move. It glistened with a thin line of dried blood, just an outline of the scar. He leaned closer, pressing into the wound carefully. "No sign of infection. Excellent. Any pain when I touch it?"

"No pain, but I can feel the staples pressing in."

"Let's get those out right now." He reached for a device that looked much too small for the job, like a nail clipper in a pedicurist's booth. He picked and yanked his way up the line, digging out each staple in turn. He was quick and efficient, finishing his work before Patrick even registered the strangeness of how it felt: like sewing a button shallowly into him, prickly and cool; like falling onto a cactus length-wise. The scar itched, releasing itself with each tug.

"It's holding together nicely," Doctor Blatt said. "Healing right up. Can't even tell it's been closed and re-opened so many times."

The appointment was over before he knew it, couldn't have lasted more than ten or fifteen minutes. He was dismissed with instructions to return in two weeks' time and a reminder about home care: not much weight on the leg, keep it dry, don't sleep or lie on that side.

"I'm gonna save that leg if it's the last thing I do," the doctor said as he left.

They had planned to stop for some food afterwards, but the soreness had grown too extreme. So Tim sped back across the bridge, a straight shot home. He laced his fingers between Patrick's, hands resting on the seat between them, as he drove. They listened to Eva Cassidy on the ride, her crystalline voice seeming to fill and embolden the space between them, seeming to reflect with perfect mimicry the almost-beautiful sadness of that waiting room. Tim sang along in a whisper, not quite sure of all the words; his lips moved unconsciously, holding their shape during the long stretches of octave climbs and falls, picking up their pace during the faster bits. His head bobbed subtly, just off the beat. And though impatient to get back home, Patrick silently watched him sing, enjoying the view.

39

At the urging of another friend, Joanie, Patrick had hired a bodyworker to visit him twice a week at home, lugging her table into the front room for a massage. He had been nervous about trying this, not sure his tender flesh would open itself enough to be touched: the scene had seemed, prognostically, too close to a surgery, him stretched out face down, eyes closed, with someone working behind him, moving everywhere between feet and head. But the first time she had come, he felt its great power, this practice that redefined *prone* away from its clinical context. That first time, the moment she laid hands on him, he had begun to heave and blow, tears of release gushing forth from him unexpectedly and without any sense of control. He had laughed then, great gusts of hysterical howling; and she, the bodyworker, Adriel, had laughed with him.

"There it comes!" she said. "There it is! Just let it out, Patrick, let it come on its own." She kneaded his back, working into him carefully but steadily.

"Oh, God. Huh! What's happening?" he chuckled up at her. "What is this?"

"It's your body talking. Happens all the time. Let it come, let it come."

He swelled and sighed, the spaces between filled with more laughter, more wails, a rainstorm in one part of the sky, sun beaming down from another.

"So much complexity in here," Adriel said. "I can feel so much inside of you. It's been held for too long, too long." She turned and pulled, fingertips dragging down from a shoulder to the small of his back. "I'm going to work on bringing it out. You might feel a different kind of pain than what you've been feeling. Try to abide it, but let me know if it's too much. OK?"

"OK," he snorted, "Yes, yes." He sighed again, transported to another kind of place, neither here nor there, neither here nor gone, some other kind of place entirely, deeply inside, but opened up, too, without boundaries. His body seemed to bloat, to expand, to unfold itself.

She had worked for two full hours on him, taking her time, unconcerned about finishing on a schedule. It was unlike anything he had ever felt before. She turned him both inward and out, wrenching the tightnesses out of him so that he felt broken and then whole, empty then full. And it *was* painful, the process—but not pain of the usual sort. It was the pain of work, of hard labor, of toiling with something small, watching it become itself, feeling the strain of making it so. It was a pain mixed intricately and insolubly with pleasure, the kind of pain that points toward a relief found only in what will come later: a long, full sleep with vivid, enlivening dreams.

Adriel was back again, now, the day before his next surgery. She came brightly into the room, dragging her table behind her. She set it up in a flash, whisking the legs open and then flipping it over, extending the ends so that he would fit. She draped a soft cotton sheet over it, smoothing it out, then gestured for him to climb on. "So tomorrow's the day, huh?" she said once he was in place.

"Tomorrow's the day."

"How are you feeling about it?"

"Oh, pretty good, I guess. Getting closer to the end, so ..."

She began oiling her hands, then his back. "*This* feels better. Your muscles here. What they carry."

"You've helped a lot."

"That's kind of you to say." She worked diligently, pressing into him. "I'm going to go easier on you today, just soften some of these knots. Open things up, get them ready for the next few days."

"OK."

"Don't want to drag *too* much out the day before the surgery."

Patrick drifted off, familiar now with how it went.

When she was done, she took another sheet and waved it out, lay it softly on top of him. "Rest there for a minute. Pick up your breaths as you can, get them going again on a regular pace. Let me know when you want to get up." He faintly heard her walk into the kitchen, heard the running water as she washed and rinsed her hands. She had lit a candle near the bed; it smelled of the sea.

He pictured himself lying there, now turned over, supine and still, eyes opening onto the ceiling. He watched this imagined set for a moment, then gradually rose, perched now on the edge of the table. Adriel had returned to the room and was sitting on the couch.

"I'll be thinking of you tomorrow, Spiderman." She had picked this nickname for him after their first meeting, when he described the ways he might have first fallen ill. She had decided the black widow bite was the most likely, or at least the most epic and interesting, of the alternatives. "I'll come back as soon as you're home again, whenever you're ready. We'll get back to work then."

He smiled blissfully at her, half-dazed.

"In the meantime," she said, "try to keep yourself relaxed. Let things flow through you without sticking. Breathe, breathe."

Deirdre flew in that night, rested and well. Jan picked her up from the airport and drove her to Patrick's flat. Joanie was waiting there with him; she had grilled scallops and made steamed rice. They sat on the couch together, talking about things.

Joanie had been a dancer, ballet, long before he knew her. She was elegant and poised, but tweaked by a long history of living in San Francisco, just enough to make her eccentric and quirkily wise. She was twenty-odd years older than he was, and had recently finished a third round of chemotherapy. She had just that day received news that all scans were clear: she was fully in remission.

"But I can't shake the chemo-brain," she said. "I'm even loopier than before. Forget things, can't find things, you know, can't remember people's names when I've known them for years."

"Ouch," Patrick said. "That must be awful."

"Oh, no, on the contrary. It's not awful at all. It's amazing. Like I have a license to be forgetful. Seriously, Patrick, I feel completely free, set loose from the business of keeping track of everything."

Patrick laughed at this.

"Like, who *cares* if I locked the door when I left? Who *cares* if I washed the dishes twice? Who really cares? What does it matter?"

"It doesn't, I guess. Not in the scheme of things."

"No, it doesn't. Not a whit. And what *is* 'the scheme of things' anyway? You know? What *matters*, in the end? *My* scheme of things, right now, is that I am here, and you are here, and we are both here together, in this place, eating this food."

"Yes we are."

"It's like, the chemo-brain has freed me from worrying about anything else, from even *remembering* anything else." She took a bite, chewed it slowly. "I like that. I really do. Feels fuller somehow." She thought for a moment. "And I can still feel them there, those split cells. They're still a part of me, you know. Remission or not."

"What do you mean?"

"I don't know, it's like, they're *with* me still. Sometimes it's like they can talk to me, whisper things in my head. Little reminders. Not threats, like little proverbs. The other day, before the results came back, I was driving, and I had this voice just come to me, out of nowhere. 'Keep passing the open windows,' it said. Does that come from something? A movie, a book? Maybe a song?"

"I think it's from a book. I've heard it before." He tried to think. "I can't remember which one—I read it a long time ago, I think. Maybe in high school."

" 'Keep passing the open windows,' right out of the blue. Pushing me forward. Like, 'don't jump! Whatever you do, don't jump!' "

Patrick laughed, and Joanie laughed too.

They had left the main door open, screen door closed, letting the cool wind through. In the distance, they heard some car doors close, Jan's voice calling faintly, "Need help with the bags?"

"No thanks, I've got them," Deirdre said. They listened as footsteps climbed the stairs and grew louder as the two approached.

"I'll just clean this up," Joanie said, taking both plates and the flatware into the kitchen.

It was a happy reunion, everyone hugging and smiling, small talk about travel, plans for the next morning. Deirdre lingered over Patrick, looking at his full length, fixing his hair. "You look great, son," she said.

"I feel pretty great. Joanie made scallops."

Deirdre checked her watch. "Are you done eating? It's almost six. No more food tonight, right?"

They all sat together for hours, talking and playing cards. Joanie and Jan stayed until ten, then quickly packed up and went, leaving Patrick with pecks on the cheek. "Good luck tomorrow," they both said in unison.

"Who needs luck? I've got Deirdre," he said.

Once they had gone, Patrick and Deirdre fell back into their routine with only slight changes: she readied the bed, he brushed his teeth and washed his face; she set up the couch for herself while he packed a bag for the hospital.

"You seem more independent," she said.

"I feel that, but I have had a lot of help."

"Still. Everything looks in order, clean and managed. I didn't know what to expect."

"I've missed you, mom." He put his arms around her. "I'm glad you were able to go home. But I've missed you."

Deirdre's eyes began to cloud. "I've missed you, too."

"I don't know if I've told you how much this all means to me. I don't know that I'd ever be able to tell you, how grateful I am."

"Can't imagine it any other way, Patrick."

"I know, but it can't be easy. Seeing me like this. Doing so much for me, knowing I haven't been able to do it myself. It can't be easy."

"I just wish I could give you my eyes."

This startled him. He pulled back, looked at her closely. "Your *eyes*? What do you mean?"

She sniffed twice, looked at the floor. "I went to see a few doctors back home. Eye doctors. I asked if there was any way for me to donate my eyes to you, replace yours with mine."

"Mom. You can't be serious."

"Why not?"

"Oh, mom. Please don't think that way. Like you need to give more. Please, please stop thinking that way."

"I just feel so bad. Your eyes, what you do with them. You need them more than I do." She was very near the edge of weeping now, overcome. She'd been holding this back for a while, and now that it was out she could hear how ridiculous it sounded, knew it for what it was: a helplessness, a futility, a hopelessness, a feeling she could not bear.

"And anyway, my eyes, mom, they're doing better. Or I'm getting used to them, or both. Really. Doctor Straddler even says I'll drive again, remember?"

"I remember." She held herself back, careful not to tip over to the other side: the sobbing, the desperation. She kept herself composed, best as she could. "I remember."

"When this is all over, you won't even know anything's different about them." He squeezed her again.

"We'd better hit the sack," she said. "Early day tomorrow."

It happened so fast, the following morning: they were up and dressed, in the car and across the bridge, waiting in pre-op before the sun even came up. He'd been scrubbed with iodine at the wound, the burnt orange spreading across his waist and down the thigh. Lorazepam absorbed, he was floating three feet above the bed, nothing touching him, nothing at all. A blue paper shower cap pulled his hair back, kept it hidden and in place. Deirdre sat next to him, reading her notes from the previous surgery, making sure everything went the same way.

Maria came round the curtain, "There he is! How are you feeling?"

"Not feeling much right now, actually. Sort of just drifting."

"Ha-ha, yes. Let's keep that going, OK?" She pushed something new into the IV line, and he faded further, a pleasurable wave rolling over him.

"Ah—I could stay here forever," he said, softening further than he knew he could.

"I'm gonna try to make sure that doesn't happen, Patrick," Maria said, turning to smile at Deirdre. "We're ready for you back there. I'll take you in. Say goodbye to your mother."

" 'Goodbye to your mother.' " He grinned clownishly, teeth together.

Deirdre laughed. "See you in a while, son. Love you."

"Love you, too." And they were off, sailing towards the doors, then sailing past the sinks, then sailing into that bright other place, voices hushed and hurried, then fading away.

40

The main scar ran from north to south far off the Prime Meridian. It had been first cut back at General, its careful geography etched into flesh by Doctor Mizrahi's blade. The second, third, fourth, fifth, and now sixth scars occupied identical terrain; they were laid one on top of the other, like burial grounds on bedrock and silt below that. It helped him to think of them as separate scars, distinct in their timing, the final product—up to this point—a palimpsest of clinical trauma and surgical precision. He wondered how things looked beneath: did the tissue and muscle, the vessels and veins, line up in careful deference to that trajectory? Did they know or feel that there would be more entrances and exits through the wound? Did they care?

And there were more scars, of course, elsewhere around: what they called "depth scars," set low in his eyes. These marked the remains of both the original bacterial advance and also the surgeon's tools, needles and knives and lasers come and gone. Depth scars stretched in three dimensions, through the gel of the eyes, down into the retina beyond. They tugged and pulled, unbalancing the equalizing pressure usually found in everyday, healthy eyes.

Scars were for keeps. Some said they should be badges of honor, testaments to survival, plaques for the pain. Patrick couldn't will himself to think of them that way. They were simply too big, too prominent, too unavoidable—they pulled focus, literally and figuratively drawing the eye—and too tactile; in a word, too *there* to be a badge or testament or plaque. Those things could be silenced or put away. The scars were here to stay.

He looked at the biggest one now, there on his leg. The nurse was cleaning it, preparing it to be bandaged again. The drain was back, sticking nosily out, drawing ugly, clouded fluid into its bag. The surgery had gone well, and he would leave this place tomorrow, returning home for the third and penultimate time. He had already passed the physical therapist's exams, already climbed and descended the stairs. He leaned to his right, giving greater clearance so the nurse could tape the gauze. He held himself there, tilted up forty-five degrees, gripping the rail. When she was done he fell back, shifting himself up near the top of the bed, reaching for the pillow. It had slid out and was wedged, now, behind him. He got a purchase on it finally and pulled it back down. It was limp with overuse.

"Can I get a new one of these? This one's almost flat. Maybe two, actually, so I can prop my head up a little."

"Sure, hon, no problem." She took the pillow and disappeared into the hall, returning moments later with two fresh ones. "Sit up so I can put them behind you."

"Thank you. Oh, that's so much better. Thanks, that's perfect."

The nurse left the room, leaving him on his own. He pushed the button and closed his eyes, drifting off. After a short confusion of alternating scenes, he began to dream of a lush, tropical village, on the edge of a jungle, someplace he had lived before.

Fresh out of college, Patrick had won a research scholarship to spend time in Sri Lanka, a small teardrop of an island just off the Indian coast. He had spent a year there during a particularly virulent period in the local civil war: Tamils wanted a homeland, but the Sinhalese government wouldn't budge. He had decided to live in a large town in the mountains, just over an hour away from the capital city. It was built around a large holy shrine, the Dalida Maligawa, temple of the tooth, which stood above a small lake. It was said to house a relic of Buddha—a tooth, as the name claimed—but was somehow, despite its size, modest and unassuming in its consecration. On the far side of the lake, he would sometimes sit, watching the monks lay out their orange robes as they bathed in a shallow pool. Other times he ventured out to a university nearby, sitting to work in a dank, sparse room with others who, though they slowly grew to recognize him, seemed always surprised to find him there.

He was dreaming of wartime in a beautiful place. The roads in town, and especially down in the capital, were regularly barricaded by the police, guarded by young men bearing astonishingly large guns, stopping every car to search its cavities and undercarriage for smuggled bombs or stowed-away fugitives. The Tamils had wanted a homeland, he thought in the dream, and what is so wrong with that? A homeland—a place of one's own, a place to call home. In the dream, which had taken the shape of an actual memory for a very real trip, he was traveling to the north, past the official lines over which it was not advisable for him to cross. A friend from the village was driving: Aathesh, a Tamil man who had been born and raised in a place that no longer existed. They were stopped, at this point in the dream, by the side of a road past Anuradhapura, en route to Trincomalee. Aathesh had pulled over to show him a wide field, bordered by trees.

"This was my village," he said, pointing at the horizon.

"Where?" Patrick asked, seeing only tall grass and the trees.

"Right there. Just off the road."

"But there's nothing there, just grass."

"Yes," Aathesh said. "There is nothing there."

"Where is the village?"

"They burned it," he said. "Late one night, they burned it all down."

"Wow," Patrick said, measuring the moment. "How did you get out?"

"I ran." He turned to the left, pointed. "That way, into the trees. I hid there for two days. And then I kept running."

Patrick looked at him. "How old were you?"

"I don't know. I was very young."

"Was anyone with you?"

"No. I ran alone."

Patrick was afraid to ask: "Where was your family?"

Aathesh turned to look at him. "I told you. They burned it all down. My family too."

The drive after that was heavily laden and quiet, until they had passed the crossing with a road that shot northwest to Vavuniya.

"This land is so beautiful," Aathesh said suddenly, breaking the silence. "It has always been so beautiful. But it holds such terrible things. So many of the dead."

The dream snapped to the end of the journey: Patrick and Aathesh in a small dinghy, being taken by a handful of locals across the bay to an island for an afternoon picnic on the beach. They had caught some large fish, which they'd roast on a fire, and brought some fruit. The men carried weapons, large automatic rifles with heavy straps and extra ammunition. His blond hair gleaming in the sun, Patrick sat at the prow, watching the water speed past. They had asked him to sit up here, but he wasn't sure why. His skin was already red, ten minutes out: it was a bright, cloudless day, hot, humid. They pulled into a shallow bay, stopped the boat on the sand, and got out. The water was warm and impossibly clear. Patrick looked down as the yellow sand whirled around his feet, covering his toes.

Now on the beach, a fire going, the fish impaled on sticks propped up over the flames, the men who had brought them were suddenly rushing around, gathering their guns and disappearing behind some nearby trees. He looked around, then heard the motor of another boat. He and Aathesh sat between fire and water, looking out. A larger vessel came around from the left; the men onboard seemed to spot them and turned the boat towards the beach. They were wearing government uniforms with small, official-looking hats. All of them were armed with identical rifles. The boat drew closer, and then the engines were cut.

"What are you doing there?" A man in front shouted in Sinhala. "Who are you?"

"Just out for the day," Aathesh responded. "Cooking some fish. Visiting from Mahanuwara."

"Who's the white guy?"

"American. With the embassy. He has identification."

This seemed to calm the man, who turned and spoke briefly to the two men behind him, then turned back towards the beach. "Hope you like our city," he said in English. "Be careful here. Very dangerous nearby. War, yes? Fighting."

"Thank you," Patrick said in Sinhala. "It is very beautiful here. My friend will take care of me."

"You speak Sinhala?" the man asked, surprised.

"A little," he said, "just a little."

"Good man!" the guy said, then waved with his free hand. The engines started again, and the boat turned and disappeared around the right side of the beach.

The word Patrick had used for *friend* was from a local's vocabulary; and "friend" was a rough and uneven approximation of what it meant. He had said *machang*, an ancient word from the realm of seagoers and fisherman. It described the person who, when you go diving for deep-dwelling fish, holds the other end of the rope tied around your ankle, ensuring you do not drown. Translated literally, it means *the one who holds my rope*. Aathesh took note of this; and when the boat had gone, and the others began filtering out from behind the trees, he reached over and grabbed Patrick's arm.

"Thank you, machang. Thank you." He looked hard into Patrick's eyes, then reached to pat his back. "Now let's eat."

He had dreamt of wartime, he thought when he woke, and of friendship, and of food. He had dreamt of a nearly-empty beach, of equatorial flora and salty-sweet fruit. He had dreamt of histories of trauma, of immeasurable loss, of a child who ran because his life depended on it. He had dreamt of hiding, of danger, of near-misses. And he had dreamt of the sun, burning sharply in the sky, glinted back across the sand and the waves—and the shadows it formed, bent solicitously back behind the trees, saving them all.

Interlude

It may surprise you to learn that many artifacts of the so-called Natural World are our family's creations. We are, at base, all artists, and we take great pleasure in the objects we shape. Your scientists recently found—others, commonly dismissed as "superstitious," have known this for centuries—that when you strip a snowflake down to its core, there you will find one of our cousins, drifting gracefully and graciously down in a kind cocoon of ice. Many of the most heart-wrenching colors to be found are mixed by us, the products of a diligent chemical choreography we use to make our homes feel safe. We even work in the medium of taste: for example, wine, cheese.

Though Patrick had long been an intimate of the aesthetic domain, he had never consciously considered the arts of things. He had noticed that things could be beautiful with or without human intervention, but he had never before been aware of the deep and rigorous sense of beauty that even the most unthinking objects carry within themselves. In other words, it never occurred to him to believe that things might act upon beauty. A plant turning slowly toward the light, he thought, was pure functionality, not grace. A cave that moaned with the wind was just the physics of sound, not a song, not a cry, not a plea for someone to answer back. For humans, this can't be true. Humans are only human, you seem to believe, so long as objects are there to be used, or useful, or at the very least still.

But we work well in—and with, for this is a shared world we are in, even for those you call things—all kinds of mediums. Patrick knew this intimately: muscle, retina, bone and blood, each had been home to us; each we had crafted into something we could use; and with each we had learned to commune. We were neither ill-trained nor ill-suited for this: our family's work—especially in that strongest of all human material, bone—has an ancient heritage. It is work that pre-dates the earliest humans by millions of years. Not long ago, in the great midwest, a team uncovered the remarkably complete fossilized skeleton of one of your most beloved Jurassic beasts, one with a particularly evocative species name: it was an Allosaurus Fragilis, later tagged "Big Al." What impressed the scientists who found it was not only the skeleton's completeness, but also its tidy arrangement in the rock, and the record of trauma it contained.

From the find, paleontologists were able to cast and reconstruct not just the skeleton, upright and menacing in its fiercest forward pose, but also a likely rendering of the story of this young animal's death. Not quite an adult, Big Al had suffered numerous injurious—wounds from a fight, or perhaps (they imagined) the result of a clumsy demeanor, stumbling and tripping on boulders, gulches, and mud. Its skin had been torn, leaving space for our ancestors to get through. In some of the most well-preserved bones, parts of the beast that had been buried in sand almost immediately after it felt its final fall, are some of the earliest examples of our presence in this mode: moth-eaten both, it was; and on one small toe, middle of Big Al's pathologic right foot, a burst abscess splayed out, petrified perfectly from epochs of resting. Paleopathology, you call it: the study of prehistoric illness. Your scientists have traced it in humans, too: but always through bone. Always, always through bone. It is our most enduring medium, in every sense of that word.

Patrick had seen our imprint on bone, had tracked our movement there, in the images of scans that now filled his files. He sometimes looked at them just for their beauty, setting aside the pangs of sorrow and dread that had accompanied their original manufacture. He thought often of that word that so many doctors now had used to describe them: lace. This evoked, for him, such bright and immaculate simplicity, a language of humble splendor, a rhetoric of intimate care-filled design. He would sit immersed in lace's invocations, letting them fill him like so much nostalgia; and in that sitting, he made room for us, setting aside for a spell the unresolved and unresolvable antagonism at the heart of illness's plea.

PART VI

41

The site with the scars had been healing; he could feel it transitioning its grip, both on the surface and deeper down, where muscles seemed to clench and then relax in new and unannounced ways, giving depth to the whole. He had begun a fresh set of rotations, moving his left leg in slow circles, tracing them out on the floor below him, every time he stood. And when seated or lying down, legs extended below him, he would slowly, carefully twist them out, knees pointing to alternate sides, holding them there, then twist them back in, far as he could. Even such small-scale ranges of motion seemed to open the flow, freeing the blood to move as it should, working the skin just enough to let him know it was there.

Deirdre had left again for home, and he was spending greater stretches of time alone. Still his friends visited, mornings and night; but he had begun sleeping alone in the flat, alternating between his bed and the unfolded couch in the den. He had found that moving between them gave new life to his dreams, loosening them from certain habits they had acquired: constant repetitions of re-lived hallucinations, fragments from the past, and confused comminglings of the two. Now he dreamed freely, his mind piecing together elements of what it had encountered that day, creating unrecognizable combinations of people, places, and things: her voice, his face; this tree, that hill; a dog from last week in a park he had only just seen that day. They had become less narrative, more collage.

Spaciousness expanded in and around him, slackening the tension of recent months, granting him options again. Some days he ventured out of the flat, shuffling down to the stairs, descending them with the crutches but no one there to spot, and moving back-and-forth on the sidewalk beyond. A few times he had made it as far as the lake: four blocks that sloped gently down, which (he forgot until it was too late) meant a small climb back for the return. It was heavy work, and by the time he would arrive back to the building, he would have to ride the elevator rather than take the stairs. Sweat poured off of him, slicking his shoulders and palms, endangering his grip on the crutches' small arms. Only once did he almost fall, teetering to the left, then catching himself just in time by popping the crutch out at an angle to steady himself.

Sometimes he sat with Bobbi and Charlotte, or Jez on her couch, watching something on television, listening to music, playing with their cats. Sometimes someone would take him to lunch, or for a long drive, or to see a film. But mostly he stayed alone, enjoying the fact that no one *needed* to be around. He tried to take up knitting (someone had recommended it both to pass the time and to sharpen his vision; she left him with frizzy yarn and long wooden needles) but he grew bored with its slow progress: half a scarf, the easiest thing to make, after days and days of work. Someone else had brought him a sketch-book and pencils; but he had never been able to draw, and his halting attempts now only served to frustrate him. The sketchbook became, instead, a diary, a place for him to attempt to remember the months gradually dropping off into his rear view.

It was difficult work, remembering, and required long stretches of time unbroken by interruptions. He would begin with the smallest thing, an infini-tesimal detail—the feel of a shot, a view from his bed—and work outward from there, tracing backwards or forwards as it came. But even these streams, behind and ahead, slipped in and out of place, so that he was never quite sure how to arrange the order of things. Had the nurse come before that particular sound, or just after? Had she stroked his arm from the shoulder down, or in reverse? As the scope got bigger, the confusion got worse: which day had felt better than the day before—or had it felt worse, trending downward? The swing between progress and decline was jumbled, shambolic, confused.

But still he wrote, outlining what he could, more and more eager to get it all down. It began to take on a life of its own, this piecing-together, like group quilt-work: each dip and pull of the needle accompanied by the free flow of stories told longingly or with distress, depending on what they described. He murmured while he wrote, tangling aloud through the trickier parts by taking on the personas of others involved in each scene. He remembered by perform-ing what he could, like child's play without the "he said" or "she said" or "they said" notations, like a one-person show.

Doctor Straddler was fiddling with the dials on one of his machines, its cold steel face, shaped like an owl's, bridging the four-inch distance between them. "Looking good, Patrick. It's looking quite good. Can you look up for me, toward the ceiling?" He reached around and tugged down on Patrick's lower eyelid on the right, keeping things open so he could see in. His finger felt cold to the touch. "There is a tiny spot here, but I'm not too worried about it. Probably just a bit of swelling on the retina. We'll keep tracking it, OK?"

"OK. But everything else looks alright?"

"It does. The scars seem stable." He sat back and pulled the machine up out of the way. Patrick leaned back in the chair. "Would you like to see the images from your last angiogram?"

"Sure," Patrick said eagerly.

"They've been digitized, so let's go over to the next room. My computer's in there."

Now in that other room, the doctor sat next to Patrick, two rolling chairs huddled up over a steel table. He pulled the images up on the screen one by one, layering them on top of one another, preparing an order. "Let's get Jaime in here to help read them," he said, "since he was the one aiming and focusing the camera." He got up and stuck his head out the door, summoning a young man in a white robe, like a laboratory worker, pens stuck neatly in his breast pocket. Jaime pulled a third chair into the room and sat between them.

The images looked like aerial photography of a landscape devastated by bombs: fields of dark, tawny red with veins like rivers stretching across; they were interrupted by large, white masses, the view from above of a mushroom cloud or flattened, ashy earth. "Here are your scars," Jaime said, pointing to one of the white areas. "This is the biggest one, on the retina in your right eye. As you can see here, it covers the macula—where your central vision is produced—and reaches across the full periphery on three sides." He moved his finger along a crescent of vein-rivered red from about three to seven o'clock. "And here's the healthy part of the retina, what remains. This is where you still have vision in the right."

Patrick watched the image actively, not expecting it to reveal itself to him more than it already had, but searching for places that might indicate change. He leaned in to the screen and pointing at a tiny spot near the bottom, where the red was slightly darker than elsewhere in the field. "What's this?" he asked.

"That's the swelling I was talking about earlier," Doctor Straddler said. "The scar actually tugs on the retina, pulls in it towards itself, and this can have multiple effects. Here, I think it's pulling on one of the veins, causing it to hemorrhage, leaking fluid into the retina, which causes swelling."

Patrick learned further in, looked even more closely. "How do we stop it from leaking?"

"It should actually resolve on its own—absorb the fluid, stop the leak. If it doesn't, we'll need to do another laser surgery there, burn the vein closed. But that would result in more lost vision, so I'd like to wait to see what happens before going in that direction."

Jaime clicked to the next image. Here the picture was more complex, more variable in its geography. Smaller white spots dotted a much larger red field, scattered around. "This is the retina in your left eye," Jaime said. "As you can see, there's much more healthy retina here, fewer scars, and smaller. This is why your vision is relatively strong in your left eye."

"Our biggest area of concern," Doctor Straddler said, pointing at the screen, "is this scar here, just off the macula. Like the bigger scar in the right, it's tugging on the retina. The risk is the same: it could tear, or veins could begin growing through, blocking your vision and leaking fluid. But if we were to do a laser procedure here, it could obliterate your central vision in the left eye."

Patrick absorbed this news. "Which would mean I'd have none."

Doctor Straddler turned and looked at him. "That's right. That's what we *don't* want to happen. And so far, it's doing well: stable. Unchanging. Calm."

"I see," Patrick said, "OK. So let's keep it from leaking or pulling or whatever."

"Yep."

"How can I help with that?"

"Keep your blood sugar and blood pressure down."

"So far, so good."

"Yes. So far, so good. Keep it up. Stay on top of it."

"And … I mean, I know I've asked this before. But, I mean, isn't there any way of healing it, removing the scars?"

"There is not. Not yet anyway."

"What about stem cells?"

"Possibly in the future, but very far off."

"Couldn't you just scrape away the scar, let the retina regenerate itself?"

"Unfortunately not. The light-receptors underneath the retina, the cells that translate light from an image into data for your brain, have died."

"They've *died*?"

"Yes."

"And you can't replace them? From similar cells somewhere else?"

"Unfortunately, no. That's where stem cells might someday prove useful."

"But for now, nothing."

"For now, this is your vision."

"OK," Patrick said, inhaling deeply, settling himself. "OK."

"This may sound strange," the doctor said, "but it's vision you should be proud of."

Patrick looked at him. "*Proud*?"

"Yes, proud. Incredibly, despite its strength, the infection did not take everything. It left a lot for you to work with."

"But chances are, I'll be fully blind one day. Right?"

Doctor Straddler leaned back in his chair and took a deep, thoughtful breath. "Chances are, we *all* will. The thing about *your* vision is that you have this opportunity to watch it—to watch the *way* you see, and to *know* it in unusual ways—which means that you can appreciate it for what it is."

"Like my grandmother appearing in the blank spot."

The doctor smiled. "Like your grandmother in the blank spot."

That night he sat with Jan, who came with dinner, books, and a movie. They had eaten pizza, and were sitting in front of the television now, watching the film. Jan drifted off but was still awake; it was an old Italian classic, Patrick's favorite, one he had seen 100 times before—but not for months, not since long before the current situation.

As they watched the next-to-last scene—Cabiria by a cliff; Oscar unable to do the deed, then running off with her purse—Patrick said, "This part always gets me. I mean, look at her, there on the ground, kicking and sobbing. Another disappointment. An endless loop. And then, what she does after—here, watch."

Cabiria rouses herself, walks out of the trees, begins the long journey back to town, still weeping. On the road, she meets a band of youngsters playing music, dancing, riding their bikes. They surround her, a sudden pageant, coaxing her up out of her grief, until she smiles that broad smile and even begins to laugh.

"So heartbreaking," Patrick said.

"So beautiful," Jan replied. "Is it about *hope*? The story? Is it meant to be about hope? The indefatigable human spirit, and all that."

"I don't think so," Patrick said. "I don't think that's the point. I think it's about repetition, about relentless repetition—about the patterns that we keep, the patterns that keep *us*."

"Another Oscar down the road?"

"Something like that. Yes, something like that. Another Oscar down the road."

42

The patterns that keep us: it was nearly time for the final operation—for they had determined that the two temporary cement installations had done their jobs well, clearing out the bone for its eventual permanent kin. He had begun to imagine what life would be like once the date had come and gone, how he would get back on his feet both literally and figuratively. He wondered how his friendships would change, easing back into an everyday-without-crisis. He wondered how he would fill his time, no longer taken up with waiting and planning for the inevitable. What would be *inevitable* now?

The time taken up by telephone calls and letters, all to plead his case against the relentless influx of bills, had swelled so intensely that he now spent several hours, every day, on the phone with some stranger, describing again and again what had happened. He begged for relief from the bills, asked that they assume he could never pay and skip to the end of the process. He begged that someone would intervene, "writing off," as Doctor Pettle had put it, the enormous balances accruing in his name.

His insurance, in a word, ended. It simply ran out, as if it had never been there at all: the larders empty and bare. In the language of hospitals and clinics, he became *indigent* in a single instant one quiet Wednesday afternoon when the final pennies and dimes from his coverage amount ran dry, absorbed (he couldn't believe this was the last payment that would be made) by the exorbitant fees for an ambulance ride between hospitals: the first, more jarring one to General, whose billing had, for some obscure error in accounting, been delayed until then. He was astonished every time he added a sum to the tally, the long string of digits at the bottom eluding all comprehensibility. But he amused himself each time he re-ran the numbers: "I'm a millionaire," he thought, "in reverse."

No one could help on the phone. "Mister Anderson, this is your balance. If you cannot pay it, we will send your file to collections, they'll start coming after you" was a constant refrain. And yet still he called, every time a new bill arrived, insisting that he could not pay. He also wrote letters, long narrative ones, and he began to experiment with them. Originally he'd begun "To Whom It May Concern," as if this greeting might convince them of the seriousness of what came after: "My insurance has been fully depleted, and I am a student. Without a regular income, I have no way to pay this bill." He would fold the page neatly, sending it back in the windowed envelope that otherwise would transport a check.

But gradually he began to relax his formality, imagining low-paid workers in a billing office opening letter after letter like his, depositing them promptly in a bin. "I know you are reading this in an office somewhere, and I know you can understand how ridiculous these amounts seem. I'm sure you couldn't pay them, either. Please help me. Please have mercy on me." And then, deepening the outreach of the drudge, "Hi there. I'm Patrick. I was raised in the deep south, but I live in California now. I've been through hell with this whole illness thing, and I don't know when I'll be fully recovered. Do you know what bone surgery feels like? It's horrible. I can't even walk on my own anymore. And I definitely don't have the thousands of dollars this bill is asking me to pay. So, listen, I'm really sorry about this, but there's no way I can write you a check. It would bounce. Hope you understand. Take care." He never received a reply to these missives, save the repetition of bill after bill, lined up in quick succession. Every day a new stack of three or four. And so he continued to write, day after day, one after the other, imagining a wide variety of characters who might be opening them on the other end.

"Your back is uneven," Adriel said. Patrick splayed out on the table as she began to massage. "It is compensating for the weakness in your leg; the alternate side, on the right, is stronger than the left, more tight, more pronounced. Your back has been holding you steady. It's been responsible for your balance. A real strain."

He reached his hand around to feel, arms awkwardly akimbo as he pressed his fingers into the wing muscles there. "Ah," he said, "yeah, I see what you mean. The right side is stronger."

"It's creating a lot of tension, hard on the muscle but hard on the bone, too. Do you think you could start doing some yoga stretches and holds? Emphasizing the upper left side—just to even things out."

"Once the surgery's done. I should probably get someone to help. I haven't done yoga in a long time."

"I can help you," Adriel said, "teach you a few poses to try. Once you're back from the hospital again."

"For the last time," he said, "I hope."

"Yes, for the last time, this time around." She began pulling down from his shoulders, encouraging extension, before settling in with deep kneads. "Tomorrow morning is big, Spiderman. *Huge.* You will have made it through. You will have arrived."

Patrick sighed out a long breath, pushing the air intentionally, feeling its weight, then pulling it back in through the nose.

Adriel worked steadily for almost two hours that morning, flipping him over near the end to push and pull on the other side. When she got to his feet she paid special attention, working on their intricate soles for nearly ten minutes each. This sent tingles up his spine, as if she were pressing buttons connected directly to an energy source, a fuse box or lighting board. He shivered and gasped, enjoying the feel. And when she turned to his toes, twisting and pulling each one singly from its socket, he sank further into the cool sheet below him, fully conscious of himself as a whole body, as a whole thing. His edges—the surfaces of his skin—felt neatly wrapped and complete.

Deirdre was back early that afternoon, and Robin and Tugboat Tim had come for a small late lunch, quietly marking the milestone: "It's the final day-before," Deirdre said.

"Last NPO," Patrick amended.

"Bet you're happy about that," Tim said. "I've never seen anyone *eat* as much as you. Don't know how you stay thin."

Deirdre referenced her family's genes.

"Oh, honey, you can't take credit for *everything*," Robin told her teasingly.

She smiled back at him. "Well he certainly didn't get it from his *dad*."

Tim reached under the table and squeezed Patrick's knee. "Not saying much. You feeling OK? Nervous about tomorrow?"

"I guess so, a little. Not too much. Just thinking about what it will be like afterwards."

"Did Doctor Blatt decide on the implant?" Deirdre asked. She and Patrick had been researching the materials used for these kinds of things, especially recent advancements. Patrick had developed opinions, and had asked the doctor, at a previous appointment, Deirdre in tow, when he should make the final decision.

"You won't," Doctor Blatt had replied.

"What do you mean?" Patrick and Deirdre looked at him, confused.

"*I'll* decide. Probably not until I'm in the operating room, to tell you the truth."

"Wait, shouldn't I have a say in this? Informed consent and all."

This had enraged the doctor, sending him into a brief but blazing fury. "I can't *stand* that idea," he'd said, voice peaked and pointing. "You think because you've seen some ads on television, maybe heard a story or two, and read who knows what online, you're suddenly an *expert*?"

Patrick just looked at him, stunned.

"You're *not*. You have no idea how complicated these things are. Sure, every material provides a different set of mobilities and restrictions. You *may* have ideas about which you prefer. But you know nothing about how these things work, how they fit with the bone and the joint, how well or badly they work in different bodies. *No idea*."

"OK, OK, look, I'm sorry, I didn't mean to doubt you. But couldn't we talk about them some? Couldn't you teach me some things about the options?" Patrick was trying to pave an even ground, trying to make space for himself, even an inch.

"I'll give you plenty of information about the specific kind of implant I choose," the doctor said. "I don't know how you don't get this: *I am trying to save your life* here, Patrick. And you want to get into an argument about what kind of *material* I use?" His eyes were big, angry.

"I thought we were out of the woods," Deirdre said. "I thought that's what you said, that's why we were moving ahead with the final surgery."

"Anything can happen. *Anything*." And with this final, haunting phrase, he had turned to leave the room, closing the door firmly behind him.

"No," Patrick said in response to his mother, dipping his fork down to scoop up more pasta, Robin and Tim looking at him expectantly. "He hasn't said anything else. I guess I just have to stay out of it."

"Jerk," Deirdre said. "I still don't get how he expects you not to take an interest, have opinions. You'd think they'd *want* that."

"What do you want to do when you get home this time?" Robin asked, changing the subject. "Should we start planning a party?"

"Oh, I don't know. I don't know how I'm going to feel."

"It could be for your birthday, or the beginning of summer, or Pride, or anything really."

"I think it's a good idea, Patrick," Deirdre contributed. "People want to celebrate with you."

"Let's wait and see," he said. "Remember what the doctor said. Anything can happen."

They checked into the hospital early that evening; Doctor Blatt wanted some final tests to be run, just to make sure the bone and muscle were ready for the final revision. He blew in and out of the room, still obviously annoyed at the earlier questions. "It'll be metal-on-metal, by the way," he turned and said just before he left, "since you asked before. It's the oldest and most reliable kind. We don't know enough about the longevity of the newer materials, and you're unusually young for this kind of procedure."

"OK. Thank you," was all Patrick said.

The doctor gave him a quick, chilly nod. "I'll send my team up later to talk about the rest, what all we'll do tomorrow. Get a good night's sleep. No more food."

Deirdre was reading back through her book, remembering various moments as they inflected themselves in her previous writing. "Can't believe we're finally here," she said. "Oh, Patrick," she said, suddenly choked-up, "what a long, strange trip it's been." She sat for a moment, looking at him, then gave a quick "Oh!" and reached down to pull something from her bag. "I forgot! This was in the mail today."

She handed him a small envelope, ornate but tidy handwriting on its face. He turned and opened it, pulling out a card made from thick, heavy stock. On its front was a wiry tree, the inked twin of the metal one sitting next to him on the bedside table. It held a single leaf, near to the top, dangling at the edge of a branch. He smiled and opened the card.

"Dear Patrick, we are thinking of you today, and sending you all of our best vibes. We know you can do this. Don't forget us, but don't let us see you in a hospital bed again." Sheila had signed first, then Aamir, the names unevenly spaced near the bottom.

He closed the card again, looking back at its front, the tree, that tiny leaf. He imagined it swaying in a breeze, clinging, desperate to remain. He imagined it staying there through winter and spring, holding on even as the snows came and covered it, even as new buds began to form and emerge, jostling but not forcing it to fall from its place there near the tip. He imagined it staying in place for whole generations of other leaves, come and gone. He imagined it holding on until the tree finally dropped, felled by age and unquenchable thirst—nestled, in the end, among the remains of all the leaves and all the trees that had fallen before.

43

Late that night, as those he now knew to be doctors explained what they would do to him the following day—explanations that were so dry, so matter-of-fact, so short on any descriptive value whatsoever that he found himself falling asleep—he was jarred out of his disorienting boredom when one of them casually began describing what remained of his thigh in the following way:

"What happens when we remove part of a bone is that it begins to return in unexpected ways." This from the same young resident as months ago, the one who had drawn his leg and then signed it, like art.

He sat up. "What do you mean, *return*? How can a bone *return*?"

The doctor, too, seemed surprised. "Well, it begins to reshape itself."

Patrick glanced to his left. "But it's *bone*. And it's *gone*. What *it* is there to *reshape*?"

The doctor was out of his depth. He stuttered as he grasped for any adjective he could find, any verb, any noun for that matter, to clarify. "It's difficult to explain!"

"Apparently so," Patrick said without thinking. And then, remembering that most doctors prefer being misunderstood to being criticized, he tried to recover: "You mean it regenerates? It grows back?"

"Well, regenerate is too strong a word. But it does start to grow. It tries to find itself. It begins experimenting."

"Sounds like a student."

"More like an artist. Like a sculptor. It starts to shape itself in unexpected ways. Sometimes out of control. You know, like cancer."

Patrick began to feel faint. "Like *cancer*? Wait. *Like* cancer, or *cancer*? What are you telling me?"

The doctor was back on stable ground. Here again was a patient looking for that calming effect that Doctors become Doctors so that they can provide. This is what they call *helping people*. He had chosen his metaphor well. He smiled. "The good news is, you don't have cancer! But your bone, the place where we cut your bone, the bone that remains, is continuing to grow. This is a good sign. It's healthy! We've cured it."

"Like a sculptor. Like sculpture."

"Like sculpture. But there's a problem. It will keep growing if we don't stop it."

"Like sculpture. Why does that sound so beautiful?"

"It isn't. We have to stop it! It can't continue to grow."

Patrick thought, then said, "How do you stop a sculptor from sculpting? That sounds so violent."

The doctor cleared his throat, impatient with his own metaphor. "This is what's going to happen. You'll go in for surgery. We'll put in the rod, the screws, the pins. We'll move you to the recovery room, wait for you to wake up. Then we'll take you right away for Radiation. We target the area, you have to lie still, we'll explain when we get there. Don't think about it now. Just rest. No food. See you in pre-op." He nodded to his colleagues, short and sharp, then nodded at Patrick, too.

And then they were gone, as abruptly as they'd appeared.

He dreamed that night of a potter whose clay refused to turn. She sat at her wheel, pressing it into compliance, pouring jar after jar of water onto the lump that she'd hoped to turn into a bowl. But no matter how drenched it was, no matter how firmly she pressed into its center, it refused to bend to her will. It was content, he thought while he dreamed, just to remain a lump, useful only unto itself. After a while, realizing that the clay would never become a bowl, could never be sold as a gift, the potter scraped it from her wheel and started to throw it away. At the last minute she reconsidered, placed it high on a shelf—out of sight—among her lesser-used tools.

Bright early light flooded the room. It was a rare occurrence: sun at this time of day, at this time of year. Usually fog kept things gloomy until mid- or late summer, when the clouds finally broke, sending everyone who lives in the city out in their short pants and sleeveless shirts, soaking up the relative warmth. He did not interpret this rare morning sun as a sign, but rather as a simple fact. The fog had just dissipated early, nothing more, nothing less.

They came and rolled him away. He was stoic, almost monastic in his meditative calm. He watched as the view swept by, willing himself to remember each of its various aspects, even the sound and the feel as the wheels bumped and glided across the linoleum tiles. He felt the soft wind of the ride, blowing up through his hair, and the short, sharp vibrations rolling up through the bed. He mapped their travel, knew that they were passing each room without looking, then the slow turn and shift as they pulled him into the lift. The doors closed, and he listened for the dings of each floor, then waited for the final slow of the descent. The elevator settled near the base of its shaft, and the doors opened one final time. Here was the hall to the pre-operative suite. Here were the doors that opened on their own. Here were the thin gauze curtains draped in small quadrants, here the sounds of waiting, here the little machines buckled into place, temporarily hooked up to measure anxiety, panic, concern.

And then the feel of the meds, pushed in to keep him steady as the moment approached. His mother standing beside the bed. A nurse to reassure them both. The doctor, come to say "It's time, it's nearly time," and then the brisk speeding up of events, minutes rolling past more quickly now, more sure of their aim, falling away faster still, and then another softening shot, and then rolling again, the doors, the sinks, the blast of cold air, and the light, that overpowering light, the last indication that he was slipping further and further away.

"Patrick. It's time. I need you to wake up, Patrick. It's time." He became vaguely aware of a man standing over him, holding his hand. He felt the rough drag in his throat—"I must remember to ask," he thought, "what that feeling is; I must remember to ask"—as the man squeezed harder, urging him up and out of his sleep. "Are you with me? It's time. I need you to wake up. We need to go straight to Radiation."

No water this time; no long, slow duration as he slowly came to; no grace in the emergence. They simply popped him up, out of the blank, and then once they knew he was at a minimal threshold for being-awake, they rolled him away again. "It's different this time," he thought. "Why?"

The radiation room was deeper down, a sub-basement, which seemed mournfully familiar: long, wide halls and broad spaces where massive machines held court, and smaller booths nearby, windows stuck plum in their middles, providing a safe view for those huddled there. He was pushed into a dark, cavernous place, slate-gray, a spotlight aimed down at a platform over which a machine craned. It had a round face, or seemed to, about four feet across, with a square window, pointed at an angle towards the long, bench-like bed below.

"We're going to move you over now," someone said, and he felt himself being lifted and turned, then placed down on the bed. He was too disoriented to know if this brought any pain, and lay limp, staring at the round face and its large, square eye. "Are you comfortable there?"

"I don't know," he said, slurring his words.

"You're going to have to remain completely still—no movement at all. So make sure you're in a position you can hold."

Slowly, painstakingly: "I think it is fine for me to be like this." Once he had said this, he thought how awkward his phrasing had sounded. "I think I'm fine here," he tried again.

"Good. The treatment won't take long. Once we have the beam aimed, you need to remain extremely still. This is very important. Completely still. OK?"

"Yeah."

"After the first round, I'll reposition you and repeat the procedure. And then you're done."

"Yeah."

"This is radiation, so it's very important you lie very still."

"Will it ..." he trailed off, closing his eyes.

"What? Will it *what*?"

"Oh—will it hurt?"

"You shouldn't feel anything except maybe a slight warming in the area."

"Warming."

"Yes."

He drifted off again.

"Patrick? Stay awake for this, OK? Focus on holding still."

"Yeah." He opened his eyes as the technician began making adjustments to the machine and to him. "Is it—oh. Is it dangerous?" he asked.

"Yes, I guess it is. Which is why you need to remain completely still."

"Still."

"Still." Finishing up, the man walked back to the little booth, then returned. "OK, Patrick, we're ready to begin. Time to be still, OK? Stay that way until I return. Won't be long at all."

He took a deep breath in, tightening the muscles in his back, and held everything, frozen in place. He felt a large prick, like a pin but much wider—like the lance for a joist—engraving his hip, where the machine was aimed. He felt the warming, too, a sunburn moaning under a hot shower.

After a time—he had no idea how long—the man returned, "Good job, Patrick. You did very well." He began tinkering with the machine again, reaching over to turn Patrick's leg gingerly.

"You lied to me," Patrick slurred.

"I ... what? Lied?"

"It hurt," Patrick said. "I could feel it hurting, on top of the heat."

"That was probably just your imagination. It shouldn't hurt."

"What does *that* matter?" Patrick asked.

"What's that?"

"What does it matter if it was in my imagination? It still *hurt*." He felt himself making an angry face, brows crossed in caricature.

"Just like that," the man said, lifting his hand from Patrick's leg. "Hold it just like that, OK?"

"Yeah. But I'm mad at you, *mister*." He held his face in its pose—a child's indignation—as the man returned to his booth. The lance again, pointing into him, almost taunting him with its insistent pressure, like an age-old method for slow, deliberate torture.

And then it was gone. "Still mad," Patrick said to the man. "Still hurt."

"OK, Patrick, you're all done. They'll take you back up now, OK?"

"Yeah." His face began to relax. "Wait, all done? You're done?"

"All done."

They rolled him back to recovery; and by the time he had been fully awakened—the nurse back in her spot, Deirdre gazing gently down—he wondered if it had really taken place, or if maybe instead it had just been the last gasp of a dream, a hallucination, a deceitful impression of what was happening to and around him, and why.

And then he was moving again, the descent in reverse, and he willed himself to remember it this way, too: the path back to the lift, the ride to his floor, and the trip down the hall to the room. Deirdre walked behind him, and when they'd arrived she went straight to the chair to write in her book. Patrick slipped between being awake and being only half-there: not quite asleep, but not fully able to approximate presence in the room, either.

It was a long afternoon, lazy and cool, the light from outside shifting occasionally through a tangled network of shadows across the room. At times he would trace them there on the floor, or on the wall, making sense of their shapes. "What do you see in that one?" he would ask himself, and then reply, "A dog," or "a two-story house," or "some people standing around a tree." They were all angles and bends; but the way they crossed one another, flickering in and out of distinct shapes, gave them a complexity they wouldn't have had on their own.

At other times he tracked sounds, listening attentively for the shapes they took, too. Plenty of soft, murmuring voices, sometimes interrupted by a hurried tone, and wheels rolling across the floor—long and sinewy, seeming indirect in their itineraries—and the constant, symphonic interplay of the beeps and burps that the machines made: Stravinsky on speed, winding across whole octaves in a flash, never resolving into a final chord.

Now and then he forced his attention down to his hip, trying to feel it from the inside out. It seemed lighter somehow, like an unstuffed toy, less wired and wound than it had felt before. There were throbs and stings, but they came more gently, within something closer to a normal range. He didn't dare move it, afraid that even the tiniest shift would occasion fireworks and jolts within him, buckling him up and down again with their insistent pleadings. It felt wet, as it had after each of the surgeries before—but now as if there were flow: a slow-moving river instead of a lake.

He could not track time. But at some point his mother appeared above him again, looking down; and the room was dark but for the glow from a lamp; and there was a tray, bearing food. She was asking him if he wanted to sit up and eat. And so he did, the bites he was able to stomach too small for his appetite, too uncertain for his famine, too meager for his need. He chewed carefully, but he tasted nothing.

For four days he sailed across the low waves of convalescence, learning again how to stand and how to move—he could discern the difference in this implant, made for action, almost immediately—neither rising above nor dipping below the surface of what he had to do: make it to Friday, when he would be discharged. He attended to each of the doctors' visits, the nurses' directives, the therapists' cautions, with studied calm and studious heed, enforcing a physical kind of meticulousness in himself, like a dancer at the barre. The days kept a regular pace, happening in their own time, as they should; and it felt easy and safe, that sway from one moment to the next.

He was aware, too, that he was experiencing his last days-before-discharge. And so he kept notes—not like Deirdre, who recorded every instruction with a clockmaker's precision. He kept notes of a more experiential and affective sort. Like an anthropologist deep in the field, he began documenting the hospital staff's comings and goings, noting the differences in people's eccentric ways of completing identical tasks. He logged chats and conversations, not as strict transcriptions, but as impressions: "Marcus seemed out-of-sorts today, is he thinking of something else? Trouble in love? He asked me if I had comfortable sheets at home, a strange and specific thing for a nurse to ask, twice, three minutes apart, as if he wasn't really in the room." And: "Maria was all counter-balance today, dulling Blatt's edges as quick as they came."

When it was time to go, he took care to say goodbye to everyone on the floor, even if he hadn't exchanged more than a few words with them. He left thank-you cards for the nurses who had attended to him but were off-shift that afternoon. He took photographs of his room, the view from the bed in multiple directions. He tucked a small note, tidily folded, in the drawer of the bedside table, hoping the next person brought in to take his place would find it at just the right moment. And when the orderly came, ready to wheel him down to the curb, he felt the slightest tug of nostalgia, a whisper of regret that he would never—fingers crossed, touch wood—that he would never find himself here again, so familiar with every shadow and smudge on these walls that it had all come to seem, in present view, like a childhood home being listed for sale.

44

The last time he went home, cool but summery winds accompanied the car as Deirdre drove, clicking the cruise control switch off and on, off and on—an old habit she had never shaken. He watched as the trees around the hospital gradually receded, then stared as tightly packed city buildings passed him by. They were trapped, for a moment, behind a trolley, vestige of an earlier time, as it slowly dinged and shivered its way up and then down a hill, holding on to the power line that followed its path from above. He saw people huddled on street corners, waiting to cross. He watched as a man with a dog took a step into traffic, then caught himself just in time, reversing his course, backing up onto the curb. He followed their slow progression to the bridge, catching a glimpse of its span just before the first length tipped over to Yerba Buena, then rose gracefully, then fell again into the lower deck of the second half. He turned to peer at the water to his right, seeing the tall giraffes of the shipyard cranes. He saw a tiny tugboat there, skimming across the surface, and briefly wondered if it might be Tim's. And then he turned back, just in time to see the sudden maze of freeways, tangled together on the Oakland side. They wound and wove around one another, making a mess of things every morning and afternoon; but they made their own kind of sense, granting by fiat that there was no other way to articulate this particular meeting-point of so many vectors of movement.

The car hitched and bumped over cracks in the asphalt, then shot down an early exit. "I hate this traffic," Deirdre said. "I don't know how you can live with it." She took an improbable left, but was correct in her navigation, having by now become an expert in these convoluted geographies. "Do you want to stop for some coffee? Or a pizza from that place you like, for dinner later?"

"Sure. Thanks."

She edged around and through a packed turning lane, pulling up just in time to grab an available spot, right in front of the bakery. When had she become so familiar with this place, Patrick wondered. "I'll be fast," she said, yanking the emergency brake and climbing out of the car. The long awning sign hung above him: "Arizmendi Cooperative—Pizza—Bread—Morning Pastries." It had been a usual stop for him; the coffee tasted of honey even without being sweetened, and the bread was mixed, kneaded, and baked on long tables and in massive ovens just behind the counter. The daily pizza offerings ranged from the typical—tomato, fresh basil, old parmesan—to the seemingly absurd—fig, walnut, pear—but was like a delivery straight from mythical Eden, fastidiously attentive to the nature of its ingredients. He could taste the grain of the wheat, the curds of cheese, the fleshy interiors of whatever had been sliced and scattered on top.

He thought, now, of the bakery's namesake: a left-wing Spanish priest who, in the 1950s, began forming large groups of workers' cooperatives in the Basque Country. He foggily remembered a story, wasn't sure if it was true, about the priest in his youth, losing sight in his left eye, and what this enabled, pushing him into a new history: deemed unfit for fighting, he wrote instead for the daily journals of the anti-fascist rebellion. He was censured and blamed, imprisoned in preparation for the firing squad. But the case fell apart in the end, and he was released. He sought holy orders—and once they were his, he began organizing collectives, establishing free and open schools and a university, his mode of attending to the flock. He had died just a few years after Patrick was born.

Patrick thought of these things, especially the lost eye, the pivot point it occasioned. "From army to school," Patrick thought, "from warfare to work." And he wondered at how subtly fate worked: it seemed to have drawn him to this place, years ago, almost every day since, from the moment he'd arrived in this town. His first stop every morning, sometimes last stop in late afternoon, that name blazing down, haunting him in reverse, unrecognized, from the path that lay before. How strangely these itineraries work, he marveled, giving hints to the futures we find.

Deirdre returned with the pizza, a coffee, and a big bag of bread for the following day. "Not too busy in there," she said. "Don't think I've ever seen it so quiet. That baker, the one with the long black ponytail, asked how you were. Said to tell you hi."

"Kazuo," Patrick said. "His name's Kazuo."

"He has a lot of tattoos," Deirdre said in response as she started the car, checked the mirror, and backed tentatively out of the spot.

"Probably more where you can't see them," Patrick said, smiling. She turned and looked at him, briefly startled, then cracked her own smile and laughed as she drove.

"I don't want to hear about those, Patrick," she said through the hoots. "I *don't* want to hear about those."

Joanie was waiting for them back at the flat, there to help with the bags and to get things settled. Diana came, too, off the books, just to see that he was ready for the road ahead. "You know what to do," she said, "right?"

"Yeah. They drummed it into me."

"Still got your list?"

"Yes. Don't think I need it as much now."

"You will," she said. "This part can be the hardest."

"How?" he asked tentatively, not sure he wanted to know.

"You've been surrounded by people helping. Gotten used to it. But soon you'll be back on your own, muddling through. No upcoming surgery, just check-ups and a slow rebuilding. Days will stretch out ahead of you, opening up for you to fill them. It can be overwhelming. It can be hard."

"Right."

"Keep moving forward, think of travel, playing pool, and … the rest." She winked at him.

"Are you telling me I'm good to go?" he asked with a smirk.

"I'm not telling you anything. You'll know. Your body will tell you. Just remember to listen to it." She squeezed his hand, said goodbye to Deirdre and Joanie, and started to leave. "Oh," she said at the door. "One other thing. Your account with us has a pretty large balance. Insurance won't respond to our claims anymore."

He looked at his feet. "I know. I'm not sure what—"

"I made a few calls."

He looked up at her, momentarily confused.

"They're writing it off."

The days opened up ahead of him, just as Diana had said; but it took some time for him to get used to them. Each one seemed full not of possibility, but of more awakenings into the long, winding ritual of dependency his life had become. He would rise in those first few mornings and reach down to his leg, touching the hip so as to remind himself that he could not yet use it in the usual ways—a caution to trip the now-familiar habits of shifting weight, holding the left steady—"touching down," as the paperwork said, but displacing the brunt of the work to the right. But things were different now, and he had been told gradually to return to what they called *normal usage*. ("And what is 'normal' about this?" he wondered as he swung to a halting bipedal mode. "It's so *weak* on that side.")

The whole world seemed off-kilter, tilted forty-five degrees, equilibrium thrown off or redefined along a sloping plain. Ironically, the return to "normal usage" destabilized every surface across which he moved, lending uncertainty to what ought to have been a bolstered foundation. It felt wrong somehow, walking this way, uncanny and perverse—and it bewildered him, every step a quick, choppy rush.

He moved on from the walker faster than they said he should, and began grinding patterns of heavy use into the arms and brackets of the crutches. That last day in the hospital, Doctor Blatt had reasserted that he would not walk unaided again, urged him to try a chair. He had given it serious thought— wheelchairs had always been objects of great interest to him, perhaps because one of his oldest friends had used one since her early teenage years. He associated them with speed and generosity and wisdom and a probing kindness that always seemed to see right through him—and laughter, great buckets of laughter spilling out all over the floor.

But he longed too desperately for verticality, a familiar orientation, and he needed something to achieve. "I do not believe," he kept telling himself, "that things *are* as they *have* to be." And because the work was grinding and often too expansive for him even to imagine another side, this sparked his sense of duty more than it gave inspiration. He worked harder, pressing his leg to the limit of what it could take, shoring up its strengths without abandoning its weaknesses. He hobbled with pride.

And he could not bear to take them alone, the long everydays. So one bright morning, Deirdre having recently departed, he enlisted two friends to drive him down to the marina, a street fair where a rescue shelter was hosting a fundraising drive. There he found and adopted the smallest cat he had ever seen: a pound and a half of pure fluff, huge eyes staring out of it, fixated on him, like a homing device. The cat mewed and pawed, anxious to be taken from its wiry cage, and took to him immediately. On the drive home, as one of his friends wheezed and coughed vigorously in the front seat, Patrick sat in the back, cradling the cat, who had fallen asleep while purring so forcefully its body and tail shook like a tremulous hill.

"Strike one from the list," he thought to himself, stroking the cat gently from front to back. And it nestled there, somehow already sure of its place, somehow seeming aware that he *needed* to care for it, needed to tend to its wants as eagerly as it needed him.

"Izzy, get down. *Down.* No, Izzy, *no.*" The cat was arched up onto Doctor Pettle's leg as he sat on the couch, pulling with its new, still-tender claws at the hem of his pants.

Doctor Pettle laughed, reached down to let the cat sniff his fingers. "Oh, it's OK, really, it's fine. I'm a cat person, too." He smiled his soft, generous smile, gazing down with parental simplicity. "Hi there, little one. Aren't *you* a handful."

"Oh, yes, he's a handful all right. Don't let his size fool you. He's driving me up a wall."

Doctor Pettle laughed. "They'll do that. Keeping you up at night?"

"Yeah, but that's not the worst of it. He thinks the crutches are toys. I'll be trying to get from the bedroom to the kitchen, and he's convinced it's some elaborate game, racing between the points, attacking them."

"He'll get used to them. Just be careful you don't fall."

"I move at about an inch an hour. I don't want to come down on his paws." Patrick watched as the cat reached up in one final desperate plea, then raced off, chasing some tempting invisible friend. He heard a soft bump in the other room, then a frantic scratching, then silence. "He probably just fell asleep. He does that all the time."

"So," Doctor Pettle said, sitting up. "How's it going?"

"Pretty well I guess. I'm getting around."

"Blood sugar under control?"

"Yeah, it seems to be."

"Any highs or lows?"

"I'm still having some in the middle of the night. Have to get up for some food, usually around two or three."

"What kind of numbers?"

"In the middle of the night? Usually down around sixty, sometimes as low as the forties."

"That *is* low. Let's lighten up your basal insulin a bit. Take it down to twelve units a day, OK?"

"OK."

"What about during the day?"

"Sometimes a little high before lunch, one-sixty or so. But otherwise fine, hovering around a hundred."

"That's great. Your first A1C—this is really hard to believe, given the numbers you had when you first went to the hospital—is actually normal for a *non*-diabetic. Below five."

"That's a good thing?"

"It's a *very* good thing. Very unusual. Your pancreas is probably still producing a small amount of insulin, helping to regulate things, since the trauma is still relatively recent. That will change over time."

"How?"

"Typically it stops producing insulin entirely after a while."

"Dying slowly."

"In a manner of speaking, yes."

"What happens then?"

"Well, then we'll have to reassess your insulin needs. Probably increase the dosages."

"How long?"

"There's no way to know in advance. Could be a few months, maybe a year or two."

"OK. Is there any way to reverse it?"

"Sadly, no. Not at this point. They've been experimenting with beta cell replacement, but it's in the early stages. And it probably wouldn't be advisable for you to have that kind of procedure."

"Why not?"

"It comes with the same risks of rejection as in any other kind of transplant. Your immune system could begin to attack the implanted cells. People who have transplants take medication to suppress the immune system, to stop that from happening. But with you …"

"That could lead to an even greater risk of re-infection. Right?"

"Exactly."

"OK."

"But seriously, Patrick, as long as your numbers stay low, and especially with your A1C in this range, it doesn't really matter. The injections are essentially making you a non-diabetic, after a fashion."

"Got it. I'll stay on top of it."

Doctor Pettle flipped through some papers on his lap. "Looks like you're seeing Doctor Blatt again next week?"

"Yes. Mom's coming back for that appointment."

"Oh! How wonderful. How long will she be here?"

"Just a few days. She wanted to come because she knows I can't stand going back to that place, and also because I have an eye appointment the next day."

"Yes, I noticed. How *are* the eyes?"

"There's one spot Doctor Straddler is worried about, in the left eye. We'll see how it goes."

"Let me know, OK? I'd be happy to go with you if you like."

"Thank you. I think I'll be OK with mom there."

Doctor Pettle finished scanning the pages from the stack and placed them on the table. "Betsy asked if she might come visit you in a couple weeks. She wanted me to ask if that'd be alright." Betsy was Doctor Pettle's wife; she was also a physician, a pediatrician who worked in the suburbs. She had accompanied her husband two or three times when Patrick was in the hospital, had brought him books about non-western healing practices, had encouraged him to think about all the things that needed healing as part of a greater, yet-unknown whole.

"I'd like that," Patrick said.

"She has a friend coming to town, someone visiting one of the groups she works with. He's a Sufi healer, and he's coming to talk with people about blended approaches to medical crises—bringing together practices from diverse traditions. She'd like to bring him along, have him talk with you, too."

"Oh—wow, sure. I guess I need all the help I can get."

"Yes. She's found him to be very engaging, very interesting. You know, Sufism is also a mystical tradition. Like Quakerism, like Kabbalah. It has a model for enlightenment, for inspiration from the unknowable."

"Well, I'd be happy to meet with him. Really, I'll take all the help I can get."

Doctor Pettle smiled and then looked down. "There's something else I wanted to talk with you about. I'm sorry to burden you with it. But we've grown quite close over this process—*I* feel that we have, anyway—and I wanted to let you know about something that has been developing recently. I don't want you to worry."

"What is it?" Patrick watched him closely, suddenly aware again that Doctor Pettle, too, had a life to lead, one that was likely full of its own complications, its own damages, its own revolutions.

"I have bladder cancer." He said this with the same gentility with which he had said everything up to that point: soft and low, careful and calm. "It isn't new; I had my first diagnosis a number of years ago, and went through a long treatment. But this is one of those cancers that is very likely to recur—remissions don't typically last all that long. And it's back again, now."

"Oh my God, Doctor Pettle, I am so sorry. Oh—oh, what terrible news. I am so sorry." He was suddenly and powerfully struck by how much he had come to depend upon this man, how fully he had begun to assume that he was a constant, unchanging figure.

"Thank you. And really, I don't want you to worry. It's not terribly painful, and I've been through the treatment before. Of course, we never know what the future holds."

"No. Oh, Doctor Pettle."

"So I'd like to begin training you, more formally, to act on your own behalf in conversations with doctors. To manage getting the care you need. I, of course, will continue to work with you, on your behalf, as long and as much as you want me to. The treatments are not terribly disruptive, so you will not be abandoned. Please remember that."

"But don't you need time away? Time to rest? I'm getting back to steady ground. You should focus on what *you're* going through."

"I am, and I will. But believe me, I want and in fact probably *need* to continue working with you, perhaps especially during the treatment. And I also want to help you become more independent in understanding your options, in tangling through doctor-speak, and in making decisions. Not just because of my cancer. Also for the long haul."

"I understand."

"Betsy will help, too."

"Is she OK? Is she worried?"

"Yes, of course, she worries. But we have both had long careers in medicine. We know how these things go, and we know that there is always an end."

"There is always an end," Patrick said, repeating these words so as to hear them again, so as to let them sink in. He felt limp, his arms and legs useless now as he sat watching the doctor's face, holding it in his mind, marking it in time.

Doctor Pettle smiled. "There is always an end."

45

He had another small scare, trifling when considered in perspective, but a scare nonetheless. He had awoken one morning to discover a small, pearl-sized pimple on the small of his back. He remembered that he had felt an itch there the day before, had made a mess of things reaching to scratch it: sitting at the small kitchen table, he had twisted to get to the spot that stung, hitting a mug full of coffee in the turn. He'd been able to get his hand around, digging his fingernails in as they rubbed, but by then the spilt coffee had spread out across the table and was dripping on the floor.

He'd mostly forgotten about the itch after he scrambled to mop up the mess; but later that afternoon it returned, more pressing now, and spreading out from the core so that the tingling now reached almost around to his side. He'd twisted and reached again, and scratched for a good minute or so to relieve the pain. And then he'd forgotten it again. But now, the next morning, a small, fiery boil poked up through the skin. He looked at it through the mirror, holding on to the sink so as to give himself leverage for the turn. There it was, angry and hot, a full three-inch circumference of red surrounding it.

He immediately went to the phone and called Doctor Pettle. Betsy answered in her low, echoing voice, barely audible. "Hi, Patrick! What a treat! Bob is out running errands. Is everything OK?"

He described the situation, having taken the phone back into the bathroom, looking at his back through the mirror again.

"Ah, yes. OK. This will happen from time to time. You'll need to wash your hands constantly, especially when you've scratched—and, yes, try not to scratch, if you can stand it. Did Bob give you some mupirocin? ... Go ahead, I'll wait."

He went through the cabinet above the sink, tilted through the medicine bottles, craning to see in the back. "Oh—yes, here it is. A little white tube."

"Yes, good. You'll want to wash the area, if you can, with regular soap. Then dry it with something you can throw away, a paper towel or something. Cover the area with the ointment, twice a day for seven days. And bandage it loosely, covering the boil itself. A regular plaster should do the trick."

"OK."

"You'll also need to strip your bed, wash the sheets, your clothes, and whatever towels you've used in very hot water. You shouldn't need to do that again if the bandage is secure enough; but if you want to be extra safe, do the same thing tomorrow—very hot water. The boil should go down within a couple days, but don't stop using the salve. Twice a day, a full seven days."

"Got it. Thank you."

"That's very important. Mupirocin is a powerful antibiotic, and we don't want resistances developing. Use it for the full seven days, OK?"

"Yes. I will."

It gave him a shock, so quick the return. He followed Betsy's directions carefully, thinking them through along the way, ticking them off a checklist he had made. Once he had the bandage on, he felt for it constantly, ensuring it had not pulled away or fallen off.

When Deirdre got in, later that day, he showed her the spot, lifting the plaster's edge just enough to give her a peek. "Oh, it's small," she said. "Remember when you were first at the hospital—well, no, right, of course you wouldn't. There was a point when you were covered in these. All over your back and legs, some even up on your neck. But they were huge—four or five times as big."

"I don't remember."

"You were pretty out of it. But when you'd wake up, when they were there, you'd howl at them, scratching furiously. They had to tie your hands to the bed at one point, keep you from pulling your own skin off."

"How is it," Patrick said, "that you can still tell me stories like this, and me not recognize them? There've been so *many* already. I thought I'd heard all of it, or *most* anyway."

"A lot happened," said Deirdre. "It was constant. There wasn't a single moment, those first few weeks, when there wasn't *something* going on."

"My God," Patrick said. "Like a building collapsing, brick after brick, never-ending."

"Do you remember," Deirdre began, pausing to get it right, "do you remember the night we stood you up for the first time? In the first hospital. Must have been a week into it."

"I don't think so." He thought, and looked like he was thinking. "No, I don't think so."

"We had gotten you out of bed, and there you were standing on your own two feet, just standing there. You were frozen in place, staring in front of you, your eyes huge, like you were surprised about something. Sheila was there, she's the one who'd suggested we try, and she was holding your arm for a while, steadying you."

"I don't remember that."

"And then she just let go—she was standing back a few feet then, and her hand just let go of you, and we all watched as you just stood, looking straight in front of you. I was holding my breath."

"And then what happened?"

"We all thought, oh, wow, he's doing it, he's up—oh, this is wonderful, how wonderful, and I remember looking at Sheila, and she had just started to smile, and she looked back at me, and I started to smile too."

"Yeah?"

"And just as I'd started to breathe again, thinking you'd done it, this noise started to come out of your mouth, the loudest noise I think I've ever heard.

It started slow and then grew, this massive scream, like a siren, but worse than that—like a monster screaming, like a dragon with fire. I'd never heard anything like it. It seemed—so big, somehow, like it took up all the space."

"Oh my God," he said.

"You don't remember this?"

"Not even a little."

"Wow was it loud. People came running into the room, nurses and a doctor or two. They stopped just inside the door, everyone looked terrified."

"What did you do?"

"Me? I couldn't move. I was stuck."

"What about Sheila?"

"Oh, as usual, she took care of it. Lifted you straight off the ground, placed you back in the bed. Got a syringe, gave you something to put you out. You were still screaming from the bed, like one long wail—I couldn't tell if you were even breathing at all—and then it just gradually died, like it was fading away, like it was coming from something that was getting further and further away." She looked at her lap, shook her head slowly. "I tell you what, there were times like that when I didn't even know if you were *you* anymore. It was like a demon or something had just—taken over." She looked back at him. "That look in your eyes. I will never forget it. Couldn't see you in there anymore. Seems like a lifetime ago now." She looked back at her lap. "Anyway ..."

"Yeah, anyway."

She smiled up at him. "Anyway, this one is small. They did say you might get them from time to time. You washed the sheets?"

"Yeah."

"And the towels, and your clothes?"

"Yep."

"Good. That's all you can do, just wash everything—and keep putting that stuff on it." Izzy came tearing around the corner just then, chasing an invisible other. Deirdre leapt out of his way; she didn't trust cats, and was mildly allergic. "That *thing*," she said, "had better calm down when it's time for bed."

He had given her his room, and slept on the couch so that the cat would leave her alone. He noticed in the morning, right after getting up, that the bed was perfectly made—all wrinkles banished, as if it hadn't been slept in at all. Once, awake in the middle of the night and mildly disoriented after going to the bathroom, he pushed the door open, catching sight of her then: she was packed into the tiniest space on the bed, as if she had been compacted. He wondered if she preferred smaller spaces, if they felt safer to her, or if it was just her nature to fold herself up into her slightest possible form. She slept on her side, knees tucked up, arms folded together in front of her head, like the perfect model of a person sleeping, just so.

Two mornings after she had arrived, they readied themselves for the appointment with Doctor Blatt, packing up a small bag just in case there was another long wait; Patrick had learned in the last few months that his office *always* ran at least an hour behind. They had some snacks, bottles of water, Deirdre's notebook, a file of papers, and some things to read while waiting.

But this time, incredibly, they were ushered into a room almost as soon as they'd arrived. Patrick had begun filling out the usual paperwork—he could do it in his sleep by now—when the woman at the desk suddenly called his name and, when he looked up, gestured to the back door, where someone stood waiting. The exam room was different from the ones he had seen before, more spacious and bright. Doctor Blatt and Maria came in together, less rushed than they usually were.

"Good morning," Doctor Blatt said. "Let's see the leg."

Patrick pulled back the gown, baring the light bandage. "Hi, Doctor Blatt. Hi, Maria." Maria smiled at him and nodded.

The doctor pulled back the gauze without responding. "Yes, good. It's healing nicely. Even the holes where the staples were are hardly visible. Any irritation around the wound?"

"Just some light itching. Nothing out of the ordinary." He had been through all of this before.

"Let's see you move."

Patrick got down from the table, then asked, "Can I get dressed first? This thing's open in the back."

"I don't really have time, Patrick. Full day today."

He turned to grab the crutches, pulled them close, and edged his way out through the door.

"Straight down then back again," Doctor Blatt instructed. "Don't think about it, just go like you normally do." Patrick did as he was told, one foot in front of the other, tracing the path down past other doors and other rooms, a few others watching him go. He was at first intensely conscious of the open gown, but eventually forgot it.

"Still insisting you'll use the crutches, huh?" Doctor Blatt asked when he was halfway back. "You could really screw things up if you fall."

"Yeah, I want to walk. I'm being careful." Deirdre stood in the doorway next to Maria, watching the doctor as he watched her son.

Doctor Blatt shrugged and tilted his head. "Fine. Looks pretty good to me."

"Now without the crutches," Maria said once he had made his way fully back, out of the blue.

Everyone turned to look at her—Doctor Blatt faster than the rest. He gave a sharp retort: "*No*, Maria. I don't want him to try that. It's misleading."

"*I* want him to try," she said, holding his gaze, then turning back to Patrick. "Give them to me. And walk slowly, all the way down, then back again." She extended her hands.

Patrick looked at Maria, then at Deirdre, then back to Maria. He shrugged and handed over the crutches. Tentatively at first, he took a step, easing down on the left leg and then quickly bringing forward the right, planting it down as quickly as he could. He paused, steadying himself, then took another, slightly more confident advance than the first. He turned and looked at Deirdre, whose eyebrows were arched, then turned back and continued that way, hesitantly but with increasing speed. When he got to the end of the hall, he turned in three small steps, more slow revolution than pivot.

"Look at me," Maria said. "Don't watch the floor." Doctor Blatt's face betrayed no emotion: he just watched. And he made his way back, each step in front of the other, a halting progression, but a progression nonetheless.

When he had reached the end of the path, back in the room, Maria squeezed his arm while the others found their seats. "Knew you could do it," she said.

"I think you'll find the crutches to be faster, less of a strain. Without them you'll have something worse than a limp, slowing you down. And the risk of falling—it's very serious, and a fall would set you back," the doctor said.

"OK," Patrick said, mind spinning with the work of it.

Doctor Blatt busied himself with paperwork; Deirdre reached to grab Maria's hand, just for a moment, to give it a clandestine squeeze. "So," she said, pulling her arm back, "what do you think? What's your prognosis for my son?"

He seemed to ignore her for a minute, then shuffled his papers together and stood up, walking out towards the hall. He paused at the door. "Ten years," he suddenly said.

"What?" Patrick asked.

"I'd give you ten years."

Patrick had come loose in the car, his face drenched with a newfound panic. "How could he *say* that? What does that *mean*?" he pleaded with the car.

"Don't listen to him, Patrick," Deirdre said. "Do not listen to him. He doesn't know what he's talking about."

"Of course he does! He's the one who fixed everything!"

"No, he isn't. He fixed your leg. That's it."

"But why would he *say* that?"

Deirdre thought for a moment, clicking the cruise control switch. "Maybe," she said, then paused before starting again. "Maybe he knows what he's like. Maybe, just maybe, he wants to give you something to work against. Someone to prove wrong."

Patrick turned to look out the window. "Maybe," he said. They drove without speaking again, Deirdre's clicking and the noise outside providing the soundtrack for the ride. They moved through the city with no resistance, no traffic slowing them down. They seemed to time every light perfectly, approaching the line just as it turned green. For once the bridge was nearly vacant, as if it had been cleared especially for them. And when Oakland rose above them, welcoming them back, Deirdre was driving as if on ice, gliding smoothly across the lanes towards the exit, then down the hill, around the lake, and finally back to the flat. "Leave the crutches in the car," she said, opening her door. "I'll get them later."

And so he pulled himself up and out of the seat, shuffling carefully into place, and began to move around toward the stairs, one step in front of the other, painstakingly slow, then sped up, climbing with all of his focus, one step and then the next, the momentum of the rehearsal pushing him on, like a sturdy tow line, one step in front of the other, heaving him home.

46

One foot in front of the other became a measure for him in those latter days, a mode to track progress. When he tried to set the crutches aside and move on his own, it looked first—and for a long while, weeks at least—more like a bridal march: step, together, step, together. But as he gradually became more stable on his feet, he was able to deviate from the dance, the "together" part of the move spaced more and more unevenly, so that it began to seem almost like a usual stride. Often his hip would bark and whine at him, still resolving into position, learning its place. And since he had tapered himself down off the pain meds, now taking only the bare minimum of the least invasive drugs, he could feel more of the strain, and came to know its eccentric twists and turns like an old route home. He was surprised to learn that movement and effort were not the only—or even the primary—rabble-rousers when it came to his pain; he would regularly feel the strain of having slept in one position, or having sat still for too long a time. If he stood without moving, testing and tweaking his balance, feeling the high arches of his feet pressing into the floor, he came to expect, after just a few moments, a particular kind of throb that would begin to swell on the outer edge of his hip, the most westerly point.

He survived public spaces—busy sidewalks were the worst—by counting his steps, and by working at the rhythm of his pace. The first few times he braved the outside world without crutches, he began marking the relation between steps in cadenced time. He moved in iambic pentameter, but he consciously aimed for free verse.

And he was exquisitely conscious, for the first time that he could remember, of others similarly positioned in the flow of ordinary life. Walking outside, if he approached or passed someone with a walker, or someone moving particularly slowly because of evident physical strain, he would match their pace and style, carefully navigating himself so as to block any unmindful others from hurrying past and potentially causing a spill. His relationship to the social pedestrian world completely shifted; he sought opportunities to staunch such flows of bodies unthinkingly rushing in all directions, gratuitous in their monotony, careless in the way they endangered the progression of others who—for whatever reason, using whatever supplemental devices—had serrated strides.

The meeting with Doctor Straddler, on the last full day of Deirdre's visit, had not gone terribly well, and had left him with a worry that expanded so that it took up more and more time and space.

"The spot," Doctor Straddler had said, "in your left eye, near the macula, has begun to flare up. Have you noticed?" He had given Patrick a piece of paper with gridded lines on it, like graph paper from a geometry class, to track the changes in his retinal performance. When he looked at it, he could see more clearly the spots, lines, and flashes that marked his visual field; the doctor had

told him to stare at a central dot, and then use a pencil to draw the miscellan-
eous figures where they appeared.

"I think I *have* noticed, actually. There's a spot, right near the center, that
seems to vibrate. But it's strange—it doesn't block the image exactly, it just kind
of blinks there, same rhythm as my pulse."

"What does it look like?"

"Hm—well, it looks sort of like something on those old magic writing
pads—you know, the child's toy. With that piece of gray film over a black
bottom page. You use a little plastic pen, a stylus, to etch something into the
gray, and it stays there, printed in the black from below, until you lift the film,
and then it disappears. It's like that, happening over and over again."

"What shape does it take?"

"Like an oval on its side, pointing towards the center."

"Yes. That's exactly what I'm seeing when I look from the outside in."

"What is it?"

"There's some leakage from a capillary, which is being pulled up towards
that scar. What you're seeing is the area of leakage, a little pool of fluid, on your
retina."

"It does go away—it's not *always* there."

"That's good. That means the retina is absorbing the fluid. But then it comes
back?"

"Yes, every so often, same shape, same flickering behavior."

"OK. I'd like for you to come back in two weeks. We'll see if it's still there.
If it is, I might need to use a small laser to burn the vein closed."

Patrick looked at him, panicked again. "Taking more vision."

"Perhaps. There are two kinds of lasers. If I need to treat that spot, I'll use
the kind least likely to cause major loss."

Patrick had sighed and nodded, his resignation dampening the mood. "OK,"
he said. "All right. I'll come back in two weeks."

"In the meantime," Doctor Straddler said, "if you notice any changes, anything at all, there or anywhere else, call me immediately. Any day, any time. If
we have to get you in same-day—or same-night—we will."

"Right."

"Chin up, Patrick. It is still a damn good eye, and your vision is still broad
and complex. Don't let this hang over you too much."

"I'll try."

But of course the spot had obsessed him, drawing him in, pulling focus,
blazing forth from its medial position. He couldn't do anything—read, watch
a screen, move around—without seeing it. Even when closing his eyes, it
winked at him from within the darkness, flickering then fading, in and out,
like a blinking hazard light, like Morse code, like a metronome tracking
andante time.

Betsy came the following week, bringing with her a tall, exuberant man wearing jeans and an untucked flannel. "This is Jeevan," she said, "visiting for a week. He is a healer. I wanted the two of you to meet." The man stood in the center of Patrick's living room, watching him appraisingly but not clinically; he smiled casually, his eyes soft but attentive.

"Hello, Patrick."

Betsy left them to talk, promising to return with food in an hour or so.

"Shall we sit outside? It is rather dark in here. Perhaps we could take two chairs with us?"

"Yes," Patrick said. "I'd like to be outside."

They moved the chairs to the broad walkway in front of the door, under the branches of a large tree planted to the side of the building. "This is a nice spot," Jeevan said, "with a nice breeze. Do you sit here often?"

"No, actually, not really. I usually go down to the lake, a few blocks away, when I want to sit outside."

"Ah, yes—the lake. I saw it on our drive in. It is lovely. It feels older than most of what surrounds it—but it is *created*, correct? Someone made it there, it wasn't just found?"

"Yes, I think so. They diverted some water, I believe, or blocked something off, to make the lake. When Oakland was young, still called Brooklyn. Nineteenth century. I believe it was the first nationally protected wildlife refuge, something like that. For birds."

"Ah, yes. Well, it is a lovely lake. But it does feel as if it would rather move. As if it would rather be a stream."

"Oh—yes, I know what you mean. It does feel too still, unnaturally still. It does, now that you mention it."

"So." Jeevan pulled a bright yellow packet of cigarettes from his breast pocket and brandished a lighter. "Do you mind if I smoke?"

"No, not at all."

Jeevan eyed him carefully as he lit the cigarette. "Would you like one? Smoke with me?"

Patrick had not tasted a cigarette for a very long time; and for some reason that he could not quite identify, he accepted. "Sure, why not."

Jeevan handed him the one he had lit, and then pulled another and lit it, too. "Smoking has a bad reputation in your country—*too* bad. Everything has its place, you know, serves a purpose. Of course there are dangers in smoking. But there are benefits too: it can calm you down, in a moment of tension. Force you to take time, if you treat it right. Everything, as they say, in moderation."

Patrick coughed lightly on his first inhale, and then was swept into a period of light-headedness, soft and pleasurable and kind. "Ah—yes, I'd forgotten how that feels. Woosh."

Jeevan smiled and took another drag. "So. Betsy has told me of your ordeal. It is extreme."

"Yes, that's one way of putting it."

"And you have survived it with grace, it seems to me. You look well."

"I feel relatively well."

"So shall we talk about difficult things?"

Patrick looked at him cautiously, tilted his head. "I suppose we could, yes."

"Good. I do not like to avoid the subject at hand."

Patrick smiled at him.

"Tell me, what was happening in your life when all of this began? What were you doing in the weeks before?"

Patrick thought for a moment, dragging on the cigarette. He exhaled slowly, enjoying the spill of dizziness it produced. "No one has asked me that. I've been working to remember the actual events, but I haven't even thought of the immediately-before." He looked at the wall next to him, trying to track things in his head. "I was writing. Spending a lot of time writing. I'm in graduate school."

"Yes. And it was early fall, no?"

"That's right. The semester had already begun." He remembered September, and October. He remembered meeting Tugboat Tim. "Someone new had come into my life. I remember being tentatively excited about him."

"I see—some *romance*. And what else, aside from him?"

Patrick thought. "I was writing a talk, for a conference back east. It was in North Carolina, where my mother's family lives. But it was in the middle of the state, in Durham. My mother's family is in the mountains, on the western edge."

"Were you planning to see them while you were there?"

"Oh—yes, I was. Actually, I think it may have been just a few days before: I had rented a car to use while there, and I changed the reservation to something I could use to drive up to the mountains. They'd had an early winter storm, and there were predictions of more snow. I needed a four-wheel drive, or I thought that I might. So I changed the rental."

"And they could not drive down to see you? Where you were planning to be?"

Patrick smiled, "Oh, no … well, I mean, I suppose they could. But I don't think they would. I mean, I'd rather see them in the mountains anyway. I love that area."

Jeevan nodded slowly, and lit a second cigarette for himself.

"Ah—wait, yes, and there was something else. My father's family—my parents are divorced—my father and his wife, my stepmother, and my siblings, they were meeting in the mountains, too. An early Thanksgiving or something. So I was planning to see them while there. I was going to drive up to see them first, I think, spend a day or two with them, and then drive over to see my mother, her sisters and brother, and my grandmother."

"Does your father still see your mother's family?"

"Oh no. No, no. It was not a happy divorce."

"I thought as much."

"No."

"Do you see them all regularly?"

"I suppose so, yes. Well, maybe not *regularly*. No, actually, not regularly, really. I try to see them about once a year—my father, my stepmother. I see my mother more often than that. I haven't seen my grandmother for a couple years, I don't think. We used to spend every Thanksgiving there, in the mountains, with her and her family. But that was long ago, when I was young. And my parents were still married. We would drive up in the family car. I loved those trips, my favorite place, my favorite time of year. And I love my grandmother. She's one of my favorite people; in fact, she's the person I always name first when people ask who my role model is. I've learned a lot from her."

"So you were planning to go back. See your mother and grandmother. And see your father too, in the same land."

"Yes, in the same land. In the mountains."

Jeevan thought for a moment. "Have you often felt …" he took a long drag from his cigarette, then breathed it out. "Have you often felt as if you were going-between?"

Patrick looked at him, slightly taken aback. "What do you mean?"

"Children of parents who lead separate lives often feel as if they are mediators, as if it is their duty to translate, or soothe, the space between."

Patrick thought about this. "Well, yes. I am the oldest child. I remember feeling some pressure there, when I was younger. To make the anger and resentment, the bitterness, between my parents, less difficult. Less pronounced."

"Did you succeed?"

Patrick thought for a longer moment. "No. I don't think I ever did."

"Children rarely do," Jeevan said, smiling at him. "But they feel that they must. It is a tangle." He smiled more deeply.

Patrick snorted a quick laugh, "A tangle. Yes, it is."

"So. You were traveling across the country for an event, an unrelated event, but were driving up to a special place for you, a kind of homeland. A safe place from childhood. And there you would drive between these two bodies, these two groupings. Your father on one hand. Your mother's family on the other."

Patrick felt as if he was catching up and catching on. "Yes—so, yes, there was probably some anxiety there. Some old feelings, very old."

"When was the last time your families visited *you*?"

Patrick felt himself losing ground again, not sure where this was turning. "Visited *me*?"

"Visited *you*. Here." He held his arms out to the side, a broad sweep.

Patrick looked at him.

"How long have you lived here?" Jeevan asked.

"In Oakland? I don't know, a little more than five years."

"And when have they come to see you in your home here?"

Patrick spoke without thinking this time. "Mom has come a few times since I moved—maybe three, four times. Maybe about once a year."

"And your father?"

"My father?"

"Your father? And his family?"

"They don't really visit me all that much. Never have, since I left home for university."

"How many times have they come, in the five or more years you have lived here?"

Patrick thought hard, then looked up and said: "Once. They were in California for some event in LA. They drove up for a couple days."

"Once. I see. And before that? When you lived elsewhere, after you had left home?"

"Not often. Probably about the same rate."

"Do they not travel?"

"Oh, they travel. They visit my siblings a couple times a year. But, you know, they all live closer. It's not as far a distance."

Jeevan looked at him, and Patrick looked back.

"But," Patrick said, "I mean, they've come since I've been sick. A few times. They've been helpful, my dad and my stepmom."

"Of course they have come. You've been very ill."

"Yes. They've come. A few times, just in the last year. A few times."

"Yes. Of course they have." He had not moved his eyes away from Patrick's face. "Of course they have."

Patrick looked at his hands, then turned and looked at the tree, then turned back to Jeevan. "Are you saying," he said, stuttering a little, "are you saying I *made* myself sick? To get my father to come to *me*?"

Jeevan's eyes were sparkling now, struck at an angle by reflected light from a nearby window. He smiled warmly, knowingly. "I am saying nothing of the kind. Things are not as simple as that. We do not just *make* ourselves sick. But it is curious, don't you think, that just before taking a trip to a place that you love, a place that occupies your memory so centrally, so nostalgically, as a place of *home*, but a place that would become, through *this* particular trip, another place where *you* were making the travel, the effort, to see *them*, and simultaneously, *you* were doing the drive, the literal drive, between your father and your mother, in a winter storm, in a four-wheel drive, through mountains—that before *this* kind of trip, to a place that you love, you fell so gravely ill that your parents, caught up in their separate lives, had no choice but to drop everything and come to *you*." He paused for a moment, drew a long breath. "It is *curious*, don't you think?"

47

Now in the latter days of physical reparation, he began to walk less gingerly, working to straighten the limp, fine-tuning his stride. He worked at invisibility, too, hiding away what had happened, packing it up and storing it so that it would not be apparent to those he did not know. He had begun experiencing that strange sort of uncanny encounter: meeting someone new, someone utterly unaware of the recent trials, and feeling the short shock of misapprehension when it became clear that this someone, like so many others, assumed he had lived a straightforward and clear trajectory, uninterrupted by clinical strife. This produced in him an unresolvable antagonism, between private and public knowledge, between intimacy and banality, between longing for recognition and hoping that no one could tell. We were with him then; and *we* knew, but he did not know that we knew.

He had returned to Doctor Straddler as planned. The spot now slightly enlarged, they had proceeded with one final surgery, horrifying in its simplicity and its speed. He sat upright in a chair, in a darkened room; and the doctor had warned him, "Stay still, Patrick. You must stay extremely still. Once I show you where to focus, you cannot move your eyes, not the tiniest of a fraction of movement. It will be difficult; it will be tempting to turn them more towards the light, almost on impulse. But you must not."

"Doctor Straddler," he said, "I'm really scared." And he had begun to weep, his final weeping.

"I know. I know. This is not easy." He allowed Patrick time to round the bend of the sobbing, then compose himself, dry himself off. "I know this is hard," he said.

And Patrick had sat back, pressing himself into the chair in an effort to freeze, rigid and clenching the vinyl arms. He eyes were wide with panic, like staring at a ghost.

"Can you see the small red light?" Doctor Straddler said.

"Yes," he said firmly, slightly too loud for their proximity, almost a yelp.

"Watch that spot. Don't look away, now—whatever it takes, do not look away."

He watched the red light, a pinprick really, the size of a period on the page. He watched it earnestly, willing it and himself to stay still. And then a bright flash of silvery green as the laser struck, reverberating out from its target in a wave across the eye, everything rolling out, a gentle swell of disappearing light, radiating away, and then—gone, all of it, in a final roll.

"The red is gone," he said frantically. "I can't find it. Doctor Straddler, I can't find it. I don't know where to look." He sat straight up, completely still, overrun throughout with paranoid paralysis.

"We're done," the doctor said. "Your retina is recovering. Give it a moment. It might be swollen for a while. You might not see anything at all in this eye."

He blinked in rapid patterns, five, then twelve, then eight. "I can't. Just a sliver through the right." He could see his hand, distorted, wavy, resting on the chair. But when he turned his eyes downward to focus on it, it disappeared, eaten up. He turned up to the ceiling, and in the same sideways crescent saw a buckled version of the doctor's face.

"Stay calm, Patrick. It's temporary, stay calm."

"Can you turn the lights on in here? I'm not sure what I can and cannot see."

"Not yet. Stay calm. Let the eye recover a bit." Doctor Straddler placed a hand on Patrick's forearm, stroking it in small circles. They sat like that, together, for about thirty minutes, the doctor drawing him out by asking him simple questions, trying to distract him in order to pass the time. He asked about his childhood, and where he had lived, and where he had traveled, and where he still wanted to go. And it had worked for a while, Patrick lost in the stories. Finally he said, "It's time. I'll get the lights."

The swelling had relaxed somewhat; but there in the center, around the spot, was a large blot, blocking everything. All focus was gone; everything was in periphery.

"This is normal. It's normal. It is exactly what I would expect after this procedure, even in an otherwise healthy retina."

"Is it permanent?" Patrick asked, eyes darting around the room in frantic leaps and shifts.

"No. We don't know yet what the final picture will be, but what you're seeing now is far from permanent. Give it a few days."

"A few *days*?"

"A few days. It will gradually recede, the swelling, and your ability to see in most of that area will return."

Patrick calmed himself, or tried. "Are you sure?"

"We are never sure. But I was able to get the vein, I hit it head-on, and with the gentler laser. You did exactly as you should; you did not flinch. I stayed away from the macula. Your vision there, it will return."

"It will return," Patrick repeated.

"It will return."

His friend Fergus was waiting to take him home. They drove in silence; with no central vision, Patrick tracked the view through the window with the side of his eyes, staring forward but watching aslant. He felt curiously calm, unbothered by the slowly fading thought that this might be his new mode of regard.

For two days he wandered around the flat, friends now called in more often again to cook, to clean, to read to him, to describe what appeared as wildly distorted images beamed out from the television. But slowly, achingly, the spot shrank, pulsing and fading like that old writing pad, gray then black then gray again, and finally resolving into full color as the swelling withdrew. On the third day, he awoke to find that things seemed very much as they had before the last laser; there was only a tiny extension, to the right of where the scar impressed itself on his visual field, only the slightest expansion in its geometry.

He began looking for lost eyes everywhere, and found them more often than not. The world was chock full of them, hidden in plain view. People he knew but had never realized were near-sighted, or far-; people with retinal tears, glass eyes and other prosthetics—all scattered around the everyday like lamp-posts, like commas, like breathing and breath. And of course Arizmendi, like countless others populating the commons, gazing down from beyond, marked in absence on that awning sign, now again a daily crossing as he muddled through and across the recovery, the reconstruction, the return.

He began to mark and describe his own visual field, especially when asked by others who started with "Can you *see* that?"—posed hesitantly and almost apologetically—and then, more interestingly, "What does it *look* like, the world, to you?" He began to find and name approximations, like: "See how, when the fog is this low, the tops of those buildings disappear? They're not *gone*, you know; they just fade into the gray. And somehow you know that they are still there, but the fog is *more* there, it's found a way to be *more* there than the buildings. Something like that," he would say. Or, when in a museum, "Like abstract expressionism and impressionism, blended together. Pollock and Renoir, painting the same canvas. Something like that."

He noted how, in looking, things began to take a different kind of place, never precise in their relative location to other things, but still undeniably *there*. Playing pool with Robin one night, late, long after most had gone home, he watched the balls bend their way across the table, even without having been given a spin. It complexified the game, made it more difficult to aim, but more interesting to shoot. He could snub blockage and obfuscation by positioning his eyes just so, strategically using the blank spots to focus more intently on his object, ignoring the rest. Without the spots, he reckoned, the field would be too full of distractions. He gave thanks, after making what felt like an accomplished double-bank shot, for the spots, for his eyes, for the warped, the fragmentary, the incomplete.

Tucked into the side of his big chair's base pad, he felt a small square of paper poking up, jabbing the underside of his thigh. "Huh," he thought, and reached to pull it out. It came quick, but a minor tear broke through its upper corner, leaving a small remainder stuck in place. He left it there, and unfolded the page: it was his list, inspired so long ago now by Diana, with a long, thin line crossing through *Adopt Cat*. He reached for a pen, and left similar lines over *Play Pool* and *Watch Olympics*. "Only one big one left," he thought, looking at *Travel*. And with fresh inspiration, he got up and went to the shelves, scanning the spines before finally finding and pulling the one he had sought: a large, old atlas he had kept since youth. He began flipping through its pages, stopping when he came to a standard projection map of the world, a globe flattened and spread out, wildly distorting relative size and actual location of each terrestrial field. "Where should I go?" he said to the book. He wanted to travel somewhere that felt like home, but somewhere he had never been before: like Alice through the mirror, rooms and scenes inverted, turned in on themselves, the familiar and yet unknown opposites of any place she had ever visited before.

48

In the afterlife of illness (for this is its long forward-trajectory, refrained in the minor key of prognosis) he began dreaming of Iceland. He had no right to these dreams, no claim upon their imagery, as his soft-pedaled connection to those far Northern Seas was limited to the usual cluster (a summer in Dublin; a year in Brighton; a handful of visits to the other Nordics). But even so, he felt somehow that he knew the geysers and rocky crags, the lava fields long ago covered in bright green. He had a sense, before he ever knew it had been built, of the enormously strange Hallgrímskirkja, a cathedral-monument to the terrible beauty of magma and heat whose clean, sparse sanctuary mapped an interiority he would recognize, when he finally sat tired and alone breathing its air, as the heart of sterility. *Sterility*—that non-reproductive quality that promises a reprieve from contagion. In hospital, it is practiced in the rituals of gloves, potions, and gauze; everywhere else, it masks its own fragility with the overwhelming stench of alcohol, tickling the nose with fantasies of untouchable propinquity.

And so, sensing this was something he was meant to do, he booked a flight to Keflavík, giving little thought to how he would fill the expanse of days, and found a place to rent in Reykjavík without even researching the various parts of town. It was a small blue house, elvish in its compact arrangement of space, four blocks from the sea. It seemed portentous, that tidy arrangement: the perfect proximity to water that stretched 250 leagues to the icy tiers of Greenland's cold shores. He went in the winter, wondering what it was like to live with four hours of twilight each on either side of four hours of day, when the sun hovered just above the horizon, leaving long shadows that cut across the routes and ways of the city's hills.

He arrived early in the morning, jet-lagged and damp from the cool-but-not-cold misty rain that surrounded him where he stood, just outside the airport terminal, looking for a taxi or bus. A complicated maze of silver rods stuck up from a grassy patch a short distance away. Small translucent triangles in simple colors hung among the slender grid, arranged to suggest an incomplete rainbow: the rods abruptly ended about 100 feet up, as if the project had been abandoned before the arc reached its highest bend. But to him it seemed perfect—like the skyscrapers disappearing into the fog, it suited his new vision, welcoming him specifically among the visitors and expatriates who arrived on flights spread scattershot throughout the day. He watched it for a while, struck by its simultaneously rough and fluent beauty, and wondered how recently it had been built. He considered taking a photograph, but thought the rain would make it difficult to come through; and so he moved on, shuffling along the deserted pavement with his bags, and eventually climbed into a small van headed downtown.

On the ride to the house, he felt distinctly as if he had shrunk to the size of a tiny doll and found himself in a miniature world. To his left, rough gray water lapped at the shore, and small boats rose and fell in oceanic rhythm, hunting fish. To his right, great mounds and dips of lava rock, covered in moss and low grass, gave the scene a mythical feel, Tolkien or Le Guin come to life. He watched as tiny houses rolled past, lit from the inside, models from a toy railroad set. He was met, at the house, by two women, around his age, who insisted on carrying his bags up the stairs and through the front door.

"We thought you would be older," the taller one, Haddý, said. "You told us you were here for a rest!" She had a full, broad smile that seemed physically to warm him.

"Ha-ha, yes, I can imagine! I've just had a difficult year and wanted a break. Sorry to mislead you."

Mirja, slightly smaller, smiled, too. She was the owner of the house. "Oh—no! We are happy to have a young man. I was worried about the stairs leading to the upper level, where the bedrooms are. I worried you might take a spill. They're very steep."

He turned and looked at the open staircase, and the louvered windows beyond. "You have a beautiful house. It's perfect, exactly what I was hoping for." There were windows on all sides of the main room, each with tiny sculptures and trinkets lined up on the sills. The walls were filled with old photographs, black-and-white, and paintings, and in one place a tapestry that reached from ceiling to floor.

"My husband is out of the country," Mirja said, "on a dig over in Nuuk. He's an archaeologist at the university here. He has many books, which you are welcome to read. My children and I are staying just a few miles away, with my sister. Let me show you the kitchen." She took him on a brief tour, stopping occasionally to explain the provenance of various objects in the room, usually a stone carving or bust.

"I work two blocks away," Haddý said, pointing to the right, "down that way. If you need anything, just call one of us." She was still smiling.

Mirja interjected suddenly, "Have you ever been to an Icelandic party?"

"Well, no, in fact, no. I haven't," he said, surprised.

"I have a feeling about you," Mirja said, narrowing her eyes.

"A feeling?"

"Yes. I do. Why don't you come to a party with us? A neighborhood party. We cook outside, just up the street. We drink together, and people sing. Sometimes there is dancing, late into the night. Icelanders know how to party."

"Sometimes too much," Haddý said.

Mirja laughed, a heaving chuckle that seemed to overtake her. "Yes, yes, sometimes too much. But you will enjoy it. Think about it, see how you feel."

"He may be too jet-lagged," Haddý cautioned.

"Well, two days from now, you know, he might wake up," Mirja said. "Think about it. And if you want to see anything around town, I can drive you. I don't mind."

"That's so kind. Thank you."

"Oh—and, listen," she said, reaching around his shoulders, drawing him in. "The Blue Lagoon is wonderful, don't misunderstand. Very beautiful. But locals don't go there. It's for tourists. If you want a hot soak, you know, a *real* one, you must go to the Sundhöll Reykjavíkur. It's just up the street, ten minutes to walk. I will draw you a map." She went for some paper and a pen while Haddý gave him a set of keys. From the kitchen, Mirja called "Do you speak Icelandic, Patrick? Can you read it?"

"No, I'm afraid not."

"Oh, we will have to change that. Send you home with a very old language. As old as the Vikings. Almost as old as the land."

Once they had gone, he unpacked his bags and set out to walk, curious to find his way. It was nearing nine-thirty in the morning; he was surprised to notice that the rain had stopped, clouds gone, making the place seem infinitely larger, more capacious. The sun was flirting with the lower edge of the horizon now, making of the sky a vast, deeply blue field, stars winking down like sequins on a ballroom gown. He locked the door behind him, careful to edge his way down the wet front stairs. He turned left, down to Frakkastígur, then left again, up the hill. There it stood, the cathedral, summoning him. He paced himself—it was a fairly steep climb—but had made his way to the crest within ten minutes. He found a bench, positioned directly opposite the intimidating entrance to the church, and sat, staring at it. The sky adjusted itself to a slightly less-dark blue, now more navy than royal.

Finally he rose and crossed the street, made his way through a patch of grass, approaching carefully, first passing a large monument to Leifur Eiríksson, its copper burned green by years of wind and rain. He paused only briefly to mark the statue's ostentation, the warm light from within the cathedral now reaching where he stepped. It was a modest door out front, less grand than one might expect. He crossed its threshold into a small foyer with collection boxes, time-tables, and brochures. He kept walking, more respectfully now, more slowly, and passed through to the sanctuary, his breath suddenly taken from him in awe of the great expanse of space, its sparse decoration, its stark loveliness. He stood for a moment that way, just watching.

He turned to his right, making his way around, and stopped at a small sculptural relief: like a thick inverted wishbone in metal, with long thin pins sticking through each leg of the form at irregular intervals, hanging at asymmetrical angles. His breathing slowed as he ogled it, perched on a podium, labeled "Píslarvottur/Martyr—Sigurjón Ólafsson—1961." He could not help but interpret it—almost in reflex—marking its resemblance to his own angled bone, the stick of his femur, doubled up and sliced through. He could not help himself; it seemed to beg for this imagined rendering, his transposition of its form into his own.

Still startled—but not painfully so—he moved on along his radial path, finding himself next facing a large sculpture of Christ, eight feet or so tall, chalky-white, and utterly pedestrian in its realism. The figure stood, not hung, one foot slightly in front of the other, arms crossed at the chest. It looked off to the right, the face riven with worry, mouth turned down in humble frown. Patrick was frozen there for a while, watching the statue as if it were just another person passed on the street. And then he turned to leave, making his way back down the hill, to the water's edge, skirting along its craggy ends, watching as the sun hedged its bets along that distant coastal line. But within an hour he would climb the hill again, unable to stay away from the towering complexity of Hallgrímskirkja. He began to feel that it resided not just in the world, but also in him—lodged firmly in the deepest, darkest abscesses, close to his core.

The city itself looked like his vision, or at least seemed to fit: fog rolled through with regular punctuality, stopped briefly to hover there, over a path, then moved on across the street and disappeared. Buildings were arranged in staccato, rarely tall, but jutting up and dropping back down in jagged patterns through town. The roads, too, were uneven: sometimes bricked or cobble-stone, other times slick and smooth; and strewn throughout were discrete sites of public art, murals and light shows and sculptures, like necessary bevels in an old window glass, fixing the corners and squares in place. He began to seek out, in particular, the iron human forms found everywhere in town, standing or sitting—sometimes together, sometimes alone—posed to suggest a wide range of affective tributes.

His favorite of these was positioned on a mortared brick walkway, near a series of steps and a small sky-blue door. The figure was orange from oxidation; it was a solitary human form, standing in a neutral position but for its shoulders, slightly slumped, and its head, hung down to face the ground. He would stand before it, each time he passed, engaged in a secret encounter, feeling—there is no other way to say this—*feeling* its slump and what he read as soft despair. The figure's right hand hung without tension or grip at its side; but the left seemed to grasp at the hip and upper thigh, the thumb stretched out just so, pressing there on the front, a slight clutch. The sculpture was named "Prospect." He felt seen by it, and known.

He spent most of his time alone. But a few days later, because Fridays are meant to be social, he left the blue house for a walk in the city, not sure where he would turn or when. He wandered down Frakkastígur to its end at an industrial frontage road, and came upon a silver sculpture—more outline than form—of a Viking ship whose simplicity stood in stark contrast to the rough intensity of the water beyond. He watched a trawling boat out on the waves, steady but for the wind, drift meaningfully from left to right toward the rocky shores below

Esja's peaks. He briefly caught a glimpse of its captain, watching the sky while he smoked, reaching in a quick bid to scratch a spot on his leg, and then turning to walk to the far side of the boat. Patrick started to shift just as a flash sparked and burned; a woman stood, camera aimed in his direction to capture the silver gleam of the sculpture.

He imagined himself now framed forever in that photograph, which would likely be forgotten not long after it was printed and, tied with others like it, stuck in a souvenir box. He could see the image, clear as the place itself, and feel the brown of its aging edges begin to creep in. Five decades hence, he thought, a granddaughter would find the old box, pause briefly on that image as she threw the photos away and carried off the box for some other use. It would make for fine storage, she would think, or a centerpiece for a display of souvenirs her grandmother had brought back from her travels. The photographs would be dumped, later that week, in an over-capacity landfill, where they would slowly decompose along with other household debris. Photographs always do.

He heaved a short sigh and turned to the left: here the magnificent Harpa concert hall, a great wall of glass windows set at fifteen degrees from vertical, the whole facade seeming to tilt, like Pisa, and slip below ground. He watched it for a while, half expecting it to move, then turned and walked back towards the house. Two blocks away, he came upon a bar too big for its paltry crowds, giving forth the sounds of a growing carousal. Surprised by its proportions, and wondering what the fuss inside might have been, he walked in and hesitantly sat down. "Hæ," the bartender said.

"Hello."

Like most Icelanders, she switched seamlessly to English. "What would you like?"

"I'm not sure. What do you think I should drink?"

"You like beer? Vodka? Wine?"

"I like scotch."

"Oh …" She turned to look at the shelves of bottles, scanning them professionally before finding her target at the very top, to the farthest left. "I think … is this? … Yes. I think we have three or four."

He was surprised to see that the three or four on hand weren't minor scotches—Laphroaig, Talisker, Oban. He pointed to the Talisker, wanting something smooth but with a pinch. "With ice?" she asked.

"No. No! *No.*"

She laughed, "OK, OK, I don't drink this, so I don't know."

He smiled. "Sorry. No, it's just that it's cold outside."

"Cold?" She seemed stunned, momentarily frozen in place. "*Cold.* This is not cold. Where are you from?"

"California."

"Ah. California." She pronounced this word in that way he liked: each syllable sharp and strung out, with the R in the midst slightly rolled. "I have been there, once."

"Where did you go?"

"San Francisco. For only a week."

"That's where I live. Well, in Oakland—just across the bay."

"San Francisco is a beautiful town, very fun. Very much like Reykjavík, in a way. Only bigger."

"Yes, a bit bigger."

"Not very many people in Iceland."

"No."

"Well. Skál!" she said, raising her own glass as he raised his.

Some time later, he sat at a small table near the front of the bar, watching the traffic pass—mostly bicycles and pedestrians, but every so often a lorry or cab. A rowdy table of men occupied another table nearby; they were drunk, and seemed to be arguing jovially. One of them reached over and tapped on Patrick's shoulder, asking him something in Icelandic.

"I'm sorry," he said, "I don't speak—"

"Ah!" the man shot back before he could finish. "An American! Are you? Or British?"

"American, yes."

"I am Njáll. Join us for a drink, will you?"

"Sure," he said, "why not. I'm Patrick." He scooted his chair back and around to face the table, hard faces glaring back at him.

"We are talking about—well, you will not know about this. Armann, here, my friend Armann, he is from the Westman Islands. *Vestmannaeyjar* in Icelandic. Do you know them?"

"Oh—I think I've heard of them. Aren't they nearby?"

"Not so far," Njáll said. "You can drive to a ferry to get there."

Armann seemed to be glaring at him in a particularly suspicious way. He did not yet speak.

"So Armann says that they are the most … well, the most difficult place to live in Iceland. He says that people who live in the Westman Islands are the hardest of all Icelanders."

"Wasn't there a volcano there?" Patrick asked. "An eruption? A big one?"

"Yes—very big. More than thirty years ago now."

"Like a modern-day Pompeii."

"Yes, ha-ha, like Pompeii. Only the people escaped. And they eventually stopped the lava flow with water piped in from the ocean."

"Really?" Patrick said. "That's incredible."

"You should go," Armann suddenly said from across the table.

"I'm sorry?"

"You should go. To Westman."

"Oh—well, yes, it sounds like an interesting place."

"But you might not survive."

"I might not—"

"You might not survive. Rough place. But you should go."

"Well … I'm only here a short time, two weeks."

"You can stay with my mother. She will feed you."

Patrick was having a difficult time understanding Armann—not because his accent was especially thick, but because his tone seemed so full of affront. "I should stay—oh. That's very kind of you. Thank you."

"You can sleep there. She will feed you. You can see the lava fields. There are many birds—puffins, many puffins."

"That's a very nice offer. Thank you."

"You will let me know."

"I will—I'm sorry?"

"You will let me know. I am here." He gestured around him, to the room. "Always here. You can find me here. I can telephone my mother, tell her to expect you. Perhaps I can even take you there."

"Thank you. I'll think about it."

"Very hard place. You will see."

"My wife is from there," Njáll added, leaning in to the table.

"No longer your wife," Armann corrected him.

"Well, OK, my ex-wife."

"She was too much for you," Armann said. Patrick looked down, embarrassed to witness this part of the conversation. There was a brief pause, and he wondered what tension might now fill the space, and whether it would lead to a fight.

"Far too much for me," Njáll finally said, breaking the silence, raising his glass, and coughing up a low, husky laugh. "Now drink! Skál!" he rejoined, bringing his tumbler so quickly into contact with Armann's that Patrick expected them both to break, shattering and spilling all over the floor.

Geysir erupted, depending on the most recent earthquake activity, several times a day. In some periods it would lie dormant, years at a stretch, its surface shimmering with low oils, steam billowing forth as from a cauldron. During these times, the staff who ran the visitor's center would sometimes pour soap flakes down its spout, spontaneously prompting it to expel boiling water, which smelled of sulfur, almost 200 meters into the air. The tourists delighted in the shows—ostensibly because of its beauty, but more secretly because they knew that it had been forced to erupt so spectacularly on their behalf.

But this was not a dormant time; and Patrick stood twenty feet away, watching it carefully until its surface rolled over on top of itself, seeming to release and then swallow again great bubbles of gas, finally giving way as the small heaves and spurts evolved into a tight stream of volcanic water high above him.

What had only just seemed a small if turbulent pool became a rocket's tail, misting away at its peak and then raining down on all who stood near. "Woah," he said. "Woah. Like a boil, just waiting to explode."

He turned and walked a way down the hill, careful to follow the cordoning ropes. Nearby, almost subtle, *Strokkur* laboriously spewed its contents more modestly but regularly every few minutes. Informally it was called "little brother"; but *strokkur* means "to churn." He watched it shoot, then edged closer, looking almost directly down into the hole. The water seemed to carry an ocean-green sheen, a glistening film, rolling and flowing across the surface. He watched as it cooled and calmed itself, receding into the hole, then slowly began to boil again, an endless cycle, a living thing.

Only miles up the road, he hiked along the sheer drops of Gullfoss falls, wary of the wet, cracked wood of the stairs and viewing decks. He had come at just the right time, the low sun echoing off the canyon walls, opening up the space between them so as to sharpen his sense of scale. It was an immaculate force, the water pushing down each level of the terraced ridges, doubling back on itself to create massive sheets of white foam, churning away at whatever life lay beneath and within them. It whistled and glowed, pushing wind that blew back across his face, hinting at the sheer power of the place.

It had appeared out of nowhere as he approached, the hills around covered in the soothing green of the softest grass he had ever felt. The only clue to its presence, just over the final down, had been a plume of mist that gathered and rolled as he walked, spreading itself out, enveloping him, then turning and drifting into nothingness again as he passed through. It had gathered in his nose and mouth, smelling and tasting of clouds. Gullfoss revealed itself slowly, seductively: first just a peek of its lowest point; then a gradual emergence into view of the second- and third-lowest shelves, spinning and spilling into one another; then what seemed like it must be the top, a spectacular arrangement of boulders, covered in rushing water and noise; and then, as he finally stepped onto the closest and most precarious viewing deck, the thing as a whole, its pristine and impeccable beauty almost unbearable to see, almost unbearable to watch as it churned and flowed.

"And here I have arrived," he thought, "in the afterlife of illness, all of it here, all of it here," reaching to hold the wooden rail worn thin and weak from years of work, dripping wet from the mists and the spray, fastened firm to the planks at his feet even as it felt that it might at any moment give way.

CODA

Another Oscar down the road: life lived in repetition. We know that story well. It rhymes with our experience, the continual merges and splits, the circlings around, the constant cycle of absorb-repel-repeat. We are all Cabirias, after a fashion.

The doctors had determined, by now, that we would always be a part of him; we could never be fully expunged. They called him a carrier, a host who would always be a host. They taught him to manage us, to understand how we work, to treat any minor eruptions with gentler salves and isolation. Breaks in the skin, a cut or a scrape, would have to be handled carefully: they feared we would enter his bloodstream again, would swim down his channels and find places to grow. But we were content where we were, on his outskirts, aside and along rather than occupying him from within, causing such pain. We felt real affection for him by now, thriving in our tiny way as he thrived in his. We were at peace.

For the most part. Occasionally some renegade few would branch out from us and make a run for it, blistering up in an angry boil. But he had learned what to do, what protocol to use, and the spot would be healed, serene again, within days. As for the rest of us, we stayed where we were. In fact we were good for him there, keeping his illness-defenses on high alert, always on the lookout for parasitic invaders. We produced an equilibrium in him. He took nothing for granted, and neither did we.

Our mother, as we have said, bequeathed to us great fortitude, and the strength of quiet movement, and the solicitude that comes from being within a group. But she is not really a mother, after all, not in the way that you use that word. (And for that matter, she is not really a she.) When we say mother, we do not mean to gesture to a single, individualized cell, an atomized one, but rather to the turns and evolutions in all the cells and all the crowds that have come before us, resolved into and as an identifiable "strain," as your scientists say. We use the word "mother" to signify not a being with her own unique name, someone pulled out of a swarm, but rather a great nurturing force that precedes and surrounds us, fostering a will-to-survive that triggers just enough change, just enough of a shift in ourselves, to dodge the threat of obliteration and make something like a home. We use it to signify work, great work—the labor of living and loving and handing-down. Our "mother," in that light, has been our deliverance; and her "lover" is the threat—of stillness and death, a menace from beyond, created or imagined so as to turn us up and inside-out before we are ready to go. Our mother is that which was there for us, always there for us, urging us forward, shoring up our defenses, offering tricks to evade the collapse. You'll pardon us for personalizing her here in these tellings; we thought it would help you to understand what it was we were trying to say, and also to see us in your own light.

But of mothers and fathers—of families organized as nuclear units, with boundaries that enforce both belonging and alterity—we have little to say. We understand that they hold importance for you, but we wonder if thinking beyond their regimented indices of identification might free you from some of the pressure you feel to conform to their tightly knitted structures of attachment. Life is lived in repetition; but there is value, too, in the deviation, the resistance, the mutation, the acting-out. Imagine a morphology of being that focuses not on cohesion, not on coherent forms and shapes of recognition, but rather on their defeat: the falling down and falling away of indignant separation, the embrace of imbrication, interdependence, sweeping sociality. Being-with is a better model for survival than standing alone.

All of this is to say: we have helped to tell you this story, Patrick, because we know that you do not remember it and so cannot tell it yourself. We have told you this story so as to release you from the tight, tangled pressure to be able to speak from the posture of illness, to be able to narrate an experience that defies the very logic of "experience." We have told you this story because you needed to hear it most of all, from someone, or -ones, you could trust. We have told you this story because it is all that we know; and because we wanted to tell it; and because otherwise it would forever be held in your sinew and bones, remembered in fractured pieces by the parts that experienced it most forcibly, but never resolving into a whole. We have told you this story because it is our story, too, and stories need to be told.

We know you are reading this long, fragmented story there where you have landed, unsure of how deeply you've been stripped, wondering how the stripping happened, and why. We know you will have flashes of remembering, some scenes summoned back like they are happening again, like they have started all over. We know some parts will seem dark, lost for good, written for and about someone else. We know you will continue to doubt yourself, to doubt us. And we know you will fear that, now the telling has been told, your body will give way, having held out just long enough to get the story right. But this is not so. Though your body has longed to tell, it has longed for other things, too. We have witnessed those longings, some silent some loud, and we hope on your behalf for the longing itself to go on. We too know the value of hunger, its pushes and pulls, and how it occupies the very bedrock of who we—all of us—are. We feel it, too.

And like us, you too will shift and change, turning into other selves, turning on the selves you've been, turning back in repetition to find and see yourself as you are, as you were, as you, like all of us, one day simply will-have-been. There is beauty in ending; there is beauty in ends. Seek to find it. For with each and every single thing, alongside the troubled but no less immaculate splendor of being, there is always an end. There is always an end.

AFTERWORD

Perched somewhere on the dark interior walls of my inferior vena cava, a tiny filter silently does its simple work: keeping watch for any debris that, solidified into a larger mass, would otherwise make the long journey from calf or thigh to lung and lodge itself there, stopping my breath. Filters like mine were made for easy insertion and a short-term stay. But the window for removal is so brief—seventy-two hours or so—and when that window drew to a close, my condition was so fragile, my mobility so negligible, that my surgeons made the calculated but risky decision to leave the filter in place. It was, I am told, a sunny Thursday in the deepest part of a San Francisco winter when the decision was made, a Thursday that became, in retrospect, a kind of wedding: my filter and I, for better or worse, made one.

When I think of my filter, imagining its little legs poking precariously into my vein, its pointy head nodding with the flow of blood, I wonder what it would tell me if it could speak. How would it describe the lightless site of its placement? How would it document the changing chemistries of my blood? How would it remember its age and slow—"slow enough," I am clinically reassured—deterioration? All of this is to say that I have come to think of my filter as a miniature anthropologist, deep in the field: it watches and waits, *in* but not *of* me, by now fluent in the rituals and dialects of my particular bodily gestalt.

As part of its ethnography, my filter represents what the professionals call *prognosis*, but what I prefer to call the afterlife of illness: the slow emergence of "survival" in a rhythm defined as much by relentless, meandering chance as by formal risk-assessment and best-guess prediction. Filters like mine are, after all, prognostic in their design and intent: they are implanted not to catch a clot already "on the move," but rather to act on the probability that future-clots may one day form and set forth on a dangerous journey. They are designed to respond to what-may-come rather than to what-is. Complicating their work, these filters are not simply silent witnesses, which is another way of saying that these filters *perform* in the very way that they are designed to protect against: over time, and especially with very long-term use, filters can *cause* clots. Prognosis is a dangerous game.

In her breathtaking essay "Living in Prognosis," anthropologist Sarah Lochlann Jain describes prognosis for those diagnosed with cancer as a complex representational space in which the present collides and colludes with a profundity of possible futures. In clinical practice, Jain writes, prognosis:

> poses both a stunningly specific (one has x percent chance of being alive in five years) and bloodlessly vague (you, yourself, will either be dead or alive) fact about the future. [It] offers a meager tease toward knowledge about cancer where there can often be little else. [It] activates terror—the shock of having harbored cancer, the fear of an unknown future seemingly presented through survival-rate numbers, the brush with a culture of death.[1]

At the same time that it operates as a kind of calculus for expectation—an ostensibly scientific dance between what-*may*-come and what-*will-have*-happened—prognosis functions primarily as a form of fantasy, like a book with multiple endings, like a film strip of photographs from different angles, like a decision tree for a committee that can't quite make up its mind. In this way, prognosis promises something that responds to the desire for certainty but can never quite fill that void. It is, in the end, a narrative, or series of narratives, into which diagnosed persons—wanting to play a role in the most vibrant and vital endings—may write themselves, at least for now.

For Jasbir Puar, this quality of prognosis—enabling storytelling about oneself in an uncertain future—serves a larger purpose than the simplistic promise of singular optimism in the face of debilitating illness or injury: it promotes and demands the eminently social project of *hope*. In concert with José Esteban Muñoz and Lisa Duggan, Puar understands hope in such conditions to be a risk "that must be taken in order to reconfigure the very forms of sociality that produce the dialectic between hope and hopelessness in which we are situated in the first place."[2] Even when, in the odds-making language of doctors and clinicians, chances for survival or recovery are very slim, prognosis always includes an escape-hatch, however minuscule, from what may otherwise appear as inevitability. And it is through that hatch, and with the gathering pull of the many others involved in one's care, that Puar suggests the promise of the social comes fully into sharp relief, in "the futurity enabled through the open materiality of bodies as a Place to Meet."[3]

The better part of prognosis—its potential to forge and nurture something like a relational hope—resembles in many ways the best kind of ethnography, which my late mentor Dwight Conquergood used to describe as nothing more or less than having intimate conversations with other people. I have this mantra inscribed on an old piece of cardboard hung above my desk; it reminds me, even when I am in the deepest throes of making sentences, that the narratives we write are above all a series of grasps towards being of, with, and among other people. Narratives describe social worlds; but they also *produce* those worlds, gathering in their sweep (we hope) a fragile collective of readers, most of whose immersions in and intentions with the narratives we make will ultimately remain unknown and unknowable to us. This is the precarious promise of narrative, especially ethnographic narrative—writing about people and groups who really exist—which has the potential to effect the very lives (and deaths) of the communities within which it is forged.

This book participates in a sub-strand of ethnography—what Carolyn Ellis and Art Bochner have called "evocative autoethnography"—in its attempt to make sense of the intense entanglements at the heart of contemporary US medical care.[4] It has distributed the power of narration to human and non-human beings in its effort both to decode and to describe how illness manifests itself in part through the radical and unwieldy undoing of narrative conventions. If, as is proposed in the Foreword, illness is a story, whose story is it to tell when the one who is ill is unable to speak? If illness is a social rather than strictly individual phenomenon, how might narrative negotiate the distribution of agency—to caregivers, surgeons, lab workers, pharmacists, and others—alongside its obligations to honor and maintain the specificity of the experience of being-ill? If narrative is a human invention, how might objects' and non-sentient beings' ways-of-knowing be translated and valued as equally informative, equally important, even equally aesthetic representations?

If autoethnography has offered a mode for portraying and sharing the experience of affect—of material emotion—in sociological and anthropological research, it has also made space in academic discourse for these kinds of questions, particularly when writing about medicalized experience. Perhaps because serious illness is such a destabilizing, disorienting crisis of being—one that treads the limits of mortality and how we confront it—autoethnography seems to have a special affinity for narratives about diagnosis, treatment, convalescence, and (to put too fine a point on it) the experience of dying. Perhaps this is because the dominant vernaculars in clinical domains—medical and social scientific description—are conventionally so dry, so stripped of subjectivity, so distant from the fleshy experience of pain, debility, and somatic trauma. As Carolyn Ellis provocatively queries in the opening pages of *Final Negotiations*, her autoethnography of the long illness and death of her partner, "Why [does] introspective data have to be hidden in our social science studies?"[5] And as she later responds: "I [cannot write] about loss without showing attachment."[6]

Feminist scholars of material culture—chiefly Donna Haraway and Karen Barad—have directed our attention to the ways in which non-sentient objects become central to the experience of subjectivity and, indeed, what it means to be human. In writing this book, I have drawn inspiration in particular from Haraway's provocative figuring of the cyborg, who

> is resolutely committed to partiality, irony, intimacy, and perversity.... The cyborg does not dream of community on the model of the organic family, this time without the oedipal project. The cyborg does not recognize the Garden of Eden; it is not made of mud and cannot dream of returning to dust. [... It is] wary of holism, but needy for connection.[7]

Similarly, Barad's invocation of what she calls "intra-action" between humans and non-humans has encouraged me to listen for the native languages of the objects and beings that are now intimately a part of me: the bacteria that thrived in my blood and tissues; the rods and pins that hold my skeleton together; and of course that tiny filter visible only as a shadow in the X-rays and sonograms performed ritually each year. Barad calls such matter "active, responsive, generative, and articulate" in the production of what we call *agency*; this book takes that argument seriously, as both the theory and the method at its core.[8]

But in addition to these more recent examples, it has been the great and too-often-forgotten autoethnographer Zora Neale Hurston who has most evocatively motivated this writing. Born in Alabama but raised in Florida, Hurston returned to her small hometown in the early 1930s to document African American folktales, rituals, and spells after training with legendary anthropologist Franz Boas at Barnard College. Describing the experience of that return, Hurston wrote that her own cultural upbringing:

> was fitting like a tight chemise. I couldn't see it for wearing it. It was only when I was off in college, away from my native surroundings, that I could see myself like somebody else and stand off and look at my garment. Then I had to have the spyglass of Anthropology to look through at that.... I didn't go back there so that the home folks could make admiration over me because I had been up North to college and come back with a diploma and a Chevrolet. I knew they were not going to pay either one of these items too much mind. I was just Lucy Hurston's daughter, Zora.... In Eatonville I knew everybody was going to help me. So below Palatka I began to feel eager to be there and I kicked the little Chevrolet right along.[9]

For me, here, now, in the afterlife of illness, it has taken a similar kind of remove and a similar kind of return to see and make sense of the experience that occasioned the imperative for this writing—in throes and convulsions, through complication and unraveling. And in the end, returning to the home of my own experience meant grappling with the radical disorientation of that home: in and out of consciousness, through countless fever dreams and hallucinations, weed-picking from the official records of my collapse. In the end, returning to that fractured home resolved itself not in the restoration of my own unified perspective on what had happened—my own studied knowing—but rather in a precarious settling-in with a fragile, sometimes contradictory sociality that would previously have been unrecognizable. And it was there, in the end, that something like hope emerged, in the afterlife of illness, in throes and convulsions, as its own kind of home.

Notes

1 Sarah Lochlann Jain, "Living in Prognosis: Toward and Elegiac Politics," *Representations* 98 (Spring, 2007): 78.
2 Jasbir K. Puar, "Prognosis Time: Towards a Geopolitics of Affect, Debility and Capacity," *Women & Performance* 19, no. 2 (2009): 163.
3 *Ibid.*, 168.
4 Arthur P. Bochner and Carolyn Ellis, *Evocative Autoethnography: Writing Lives and Telling Stories* (New York: Routledge, 2016).
5 Carolyn Ellis, *Final Negotiations: A Story of Love, Loss, and Chronic Illness* (Philadelphia: Temple University Press, 1995), 7.
6 *Ibid.*, 9.
7 Donna J. Haraway, *Simians, Cyborgs, and Women: The Reinvention of Nature* (New York: Routledge, 1991), 151.
8 Karen Barad, "Intra-actions: Interview by Adam Kleinmann," *Mousse* 34 (2012): 80.
9 Zora Neale Hurston, *Mules and Men* (New York: HarperCollins, 1935 [1990]), 1–3.

ACKNOWLEDGMENTS

This book was written in four cities over a period of ten years: in Oakland, California; San Diego, California; Vancouver, British Columbia; and Reykjavík, Iceland. I am enormously grateful to the many people who nurtured and sustained me during my time in each of those cities.

So many people have read and provided enlivening feedback on various portions of this text: Samia Abou-Samra, Morana Alac, Mona Bower, Julie Burelle, Renu Cappelli, Lisa Cartwright, Jakeya Caruthers, Giovanna Chesler, Catherine Cole, Renee Alexander Craft, Reid Davis, Dan Deforge, Jill Dolan, Page DuBois, Anne Finger, Laurel Friedman, Peter Gadol, Craig Gingrich-Philbrook, Yelena Gluzman, Brian Goldfarb, Peter Goodwin, Kevin Gotkin, Mark Griffith, Val Hartouni, Louise Hickman, Leon Hilton, Mitchum Huehls, George Iwaki, Jenefer Johnson, Georgina Kleege, Cathy Kudlick, Warren Mark Liew, Marissa Lopez, Heather Love, Lisa Lowe, John Margolis, Victoria Marks, Darrin Martin, Mazdak Mazarei, Jisha Menon, Lisa Merrill, Mara Mills, Robert Morales, Chandra Mukerji, Ciara Murphy, Joe Nugent, Yumi Pak, Peggy Phelan, Della Pollock, Ivan Ramos, Ned Randolph, Daniel Sack, David Serlin, Alan Shefsky, Kaja Silverman, Renae Skarin, Monica Stufft, Stefen Tanaka, Ernesto Tanjuan, Kalindi Vora, Michaela Walsh, Kara Wentworth, Nia Witherspoon, and Hentyle Yapp. Thanks to each of you for giving me some of your time and for the careful and thoughtful generosity of your responses.

From the moment I began talking with Hannah Shakespeare and Carolyn Ellis, it was clear that the "Writing Lives" series at Routledge would be the publishing home for this work. Since our first conversations, Hannah and Carolyn have treated this text with meticulous care and even love. My undying thanks to both of you, to the generous anonymous readers, and to everyone at

Routledge—especially the always-on-point Matt Bickerton—for helping to bring this book into the world.

To my families of origin, my chosen families, and (somewhere between the two) my academic families: thank you for claiming me as one of your own.

This book is dedicated to my mother, who gave up months of her life to be with me when I needed her most; and to Kaja Silverman, who assured me not only that I *could*, but that I *must* write this book.

INDEX

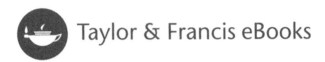

Printed in the United States
By Bookmasters